'Exquisite.'

Fearne Cotton, broadcaster, author and founder of Happy Place

'A paean to the longer-term pleasures of
staying booze-free.'

The Guardian

'*Sunshine Warm Sober* is for anyone reconsidering their
relationship with alcohol. Catherine Gray doesn't preach
or prescribe; instead, she offers humour, compassion, and
wisdom. This is the kind of book that changes lives, and
very possibly saves them.'

The Lancet Psychiatry

'A reflective, raw and riveting read. A beautiful book on
what it takes to root for yourself.'

Emma Gannon, author and Ctrl Alt Delete podcast host

'No other author writes about sober living with as much
warmth or emotional range as Catherine Gray. Her deep
insight into the subtle psychologies of drinking, and of
life, means that everything she writes is both utterly
relatable and stretches our minds. Hers is a rare wisdom.'

Dr Richard Piper, CEO of Alcohol Change UK

sunshine
warm
sober

the unexpected joy of
being sober – forever

sunshine warm sober

the unexpected joy of being sober – forever

catherine gray

ASTER*

For the world's barflies, boozehounds, hellraisers, party animals and hedonists.

Whether ex- or current, you are *my people.*

ASTER*

First published in Great Britain in 2021 by Aster, an imprint of
Octopus Publishing Group Ltd
Carmelite House
50 Victoria Embankment
London EC4Y 0DZ
www.octopusbooks.co.uk

An Hachette UK Company
www.hachette.co.uk
First published in paperback in 2022
Text copyright © Catherine Gray 2021, 2022

Distributed in the US by
Hachette Book Group
1290 Avenue of the Americas
4th and 5th Floors
New York, NY 10104

Distributed in Canada by
Canadian Manda Group
664 Annette St.
Toronto, Ontario, Canada M6S 2C8

ISBN 978-1-78325-540-5
A CIP catalogue record for this book is available from the British Library.

Printed and bound in Great Britain
10 9 8 7 6 5 4 3 2 1
Some names and identities have been changed

This FSC® label means that materials used for the product have been responsibly sourced

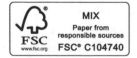

Publisher: Stephanie Jackson
Senior Editor: Pauline Bache
Editorial Assistant: Louisa Johnson
Copyeditor: Michaela Twite
Research Assistant: Kate Faithfull
Art Director: Yasia Williams
Cover Design: Mel Four
Typesetter: Jeremy Tilston at The Oak Studio
Production Manager: Caroline Alberti

CONTENTS

Preface   4

The Hooked Fish   7

Introduction   9

I: YEAR FIVE   27

II: YEAR SIX   123

III: YEAR SEVEN   201

IV: YEAR EIGHT   261

The Hooked Fish (cont'd)   262

Afterword   267

Sources   273
Index   285
Also available from Catherine Gray   290
Acknowledgements   293

EXT. GLENARIFF FOREST PARK. ANTRIM. DAY

11 JUNE 2009

CATHERINE GRAY and her father BRYAN walk through what looks like an elven glade. Lush trees overhang, steep banks are flanked with emerald moss, violet foxgloves blaze across sunspots and waterfalls crash into cola-coloured pools.

BRYAN
'So, I realised that today I am a whole 15 years sober, baby!'

CATHERINE
'Gosh, that's a long time. Well done. But isn't life a bit of a drag? Y'know, stone cold sober?'

BRYAN
'Not at all. That's propaganda. It doesn't feel like that.'
BRYAN runs up a bank to a sunspot and spins, arms wide.

BRYAN
'It feels like this! It's marvellous! Waking up not feeling as if you're inside a rhino's ass.'
CATHERINE rolls her eyes. She's restless, shifty, bored. Enough nature, already.

CATHERINE
'C'mon Julie Andrews, let's get something to eat.'

BRYAN
'No doubt you'll want several somethings to drink too.'

BRYAN is no longer spinning, The Sound of Music *style. His face ever-so-slightly crumples as he climbs down off the bank. Oh well.*

CATHERINE
'Is it a crime to have a glass of wine on my holidays?!'

BRYAN
(resigned)
'C'mon, let's get you to the pub.'
They set off down the serpentine path. Something rustles in the undergrowth. BRYAN meerkats his neck to try and see what it is. CATHERINE has zero interest.

BRYAN
'Did you know this is one of the few places in Northern Ireland you still see red squirrels?'

CATHERINE
'What pub are we going to?'

BRYAN
'There's even a red squirrel protection society.'
CATHERINE doesn't give a flying fuck.

CATHERINE
'Will we go to Johnny Joe's?'

He was right, of course. About sobriety feeling sunshine warm, rather than stony cold. But I wouldn't find that out myself for another four years.

stone cold sober: A negatively-slanted, oft-used British term to denote a lack of alcohol in your system. Something Brits heard on the regular growing up, particularly Generation X-ers and Baby Boomers. Millennials and Generation Z-ers, from my canvassing, are less aware of this phrase, which is in-ter-esting and suggests it is on its way out.

sunshine warm sober: A term I coined as a positive riposte to stone cold sober. '

Sunshine warm' encapsulates how it actually feels to be sober, once you get past the white-knuckling early days of:

'Well, it's official. I'm going to be the first person on the planet to actually die of anxiety.'

It feels beautiful, mellow, temperate and clear; like a fine summer's day.

Also, 'soft hot sober' sounded like an entirely different, naughty sort of a book.

PREFACE

'Much to learn, you still have'

Yoda

I was four years sober when I wrote *The Unexpected Joy of Being Sober*. Back then, even though I would've breathily, beatifically told you that one of my daily mottos was 'My cup is never full' (*peace sign*) as in 'there's always more to learn', secretly, I thought I'd learned *most of what I was going to* about recovering from being a raging wreckhead. Ha! What a mega-twit. If I could have a superpower, it would be hindsight in the moment.

Yoda is right. Much to learn, I still have. I am still learning about alcohol; the most glorified, reviled, celebrated, despised, manipulated, marketed and binged substance on the planet. I'm constantly surprised by new information on the enormous impact it has on our mental, physical, social, parental, sexual, familial and financial health. And I've dug up new dirt on how cunning, maddening and powerful the kingpins of the booze industry are – Big Alcohol.

But most of all, I've learned a damn sight more about how to adult as a sober, how to be happy as a teetotaller, how to create healthy relationships as a non-drinker and how to thrive as an abstainer in an alco-centric society that sometimes literally chants 'drink, drink, drink!' at us.

I'm now over seven years sober. This book is everything I've added to my never-full cup in the past three years. And no, I didn't write it because I was bored and couldn't think of a fresh topic. I wrote it because I couldn't *not* write it. There's so much more I wanted to tell you. *Needed* to tell you! It's everything I wish I'd known before going sober, or in the first 30 days, or indeed in the first four years.

My assumed reader is those who have already joined sober village. But what's that saying about assumption; that it makes an ass of you and me? That. Except it only makes an ass of me. You have a lovely ass.

While this book *is* intended as a sequel to *The Unexpected Joy of Being Sober*, thus it's ideally read after *that* book, do whatever the fuckety fuck you want. You're an adult. It's not for me to tell you what to do.

But if you do want tips, tools, tricks and takeaways on how to navigate the early days of teetotalling, *The Unexpected Joy of Being Sober* is your badger (plus the follow-up, interactive *The Unexpected Joy of Being Sober Journal*). There, you'll find the blueprints for my sober launch pad: practical tools for the first 30 days, 'what do I tell people' tips, ways to ease sober socialising, teetotal friend-finding, further reading; it's all there.

Regardless, read the books in any order you darn well please. If you like to colour outside the lines, bend the rules, do things backwards, upturn the status quo, then you're in the right place. This is the isle of rule-benders and contrarians. We used to rebel by getting spangled; now we rebel by keeping our sober heads, even when all about us are losing theirs.

I realise many of the sober-curious will read this while still drinking (literally). Welcome, my boozehound friends! Feel free to continue to send me pictures of the book + alcohol. I'm the last person to judge drinkers. It'd be rich of me to judge 'em, given I drank myself legless for 21 years and once used my teeth to open beer. Drinkers are my people.

I could conceivably be described as a teensy bit anti-alcohol these days (understatement of the century: it's hard not to be, once you start mining the reality + corruption), but I am not remotely anti-drinker.

I understand why people drink. I understand that pipe dream of perfect togetherness that you chase until the bottom of the bottle; that sprite of the ultimate night out that you chase down until you find yourself at a lock-in in Balham at 3am doing lines of coke off a cracked CD case (just me?).

No matter where you currently are in this journey, think of me as your broad on a horse who rides ahead into the fray to report back on what things – both beautiful and beastly – are awaiting you further on. Should you choose to commence, or continue, this wild, sober ride.

Whatever your intention in reading this book, whether to gawk or grow, I promise this: I'll make it as entertaining as I possibly can.

Catherine

THE HOOKED FISH

BY CATHERINE GRAY

Once upon a tide there was a fish that got caught on a hook.

The fish didn't know it was a hook. All it saw was a flash of feathers and a spin of neon, dancing through the water.

The fish stopped in front of the curiosity. It danced too, for a while. It felt spellbound, exhilarated, intoxicated by this newfound enigma.

And then, it tried to put it in its mouth, to see if it was something tasty, because that's what happens in the fish-eat-fish ocean.

Yeuch! It spat it out. Not enjoyable. But then, it tried again. And this time, something happened. It got stuck. It became twinned with the neon it-knew-not-what.

A long while passed. The night sky drew a blanket over the ocean, and stars that were already dead pushed pinpricks of ancient light through the atmosphere.

The fish decided to leave its new friend, tired of this enmeshment, but an unprecedented pain pierced. The more it tried to swim away, the more the pain skewered it.

The fish was hooked.

Until one day, the pain grew to be such, and the open ocean looked so beguiling, that the fish decided to try to free itself with all its might and smarts. It acknowledged its predicament, the existence of the hook. And then it devised a strategy to unhook.

The first unhooking plan worked for a while until – hellfire – the fish became hooked again.

Another strategy was launched.

Nope, not that one either.

Finally, after what felt like for ever, the fish heeded the lessons contained within the misfires and failed launches. It wriggled free and clear of the hook.

Joy!

It jumped, shone and somersaulted through the zero-gravity big wide blue.

But no matter how far it swam, the hook followed the fish. It feathered and flashed on the edge of its pool of vision. 'It'll go away,' thought the fish, 'just ignore it.'

Years rolled by. The unhooked fish grew safer in the knowledge that it would not be riven by that pain again. It knew now that the hook would never come closer, unless the fish went closer to it. It knew that even though the lure simmered and split, suggesting the portal to a different, better dimension, that this was all feathers and fiction; and that the fish preferred this dimension.

But still, the hook remained tauntingly at the edge of its vision.

'When', the fish asked itself. 'When will I be free of seeing this godforsaken hook, that once caused me such angst?

How will I live a happily unhooked life, if this hook is always going to be there?'

INTRODUCTION

In years dot to four of sobriety, I learned how to do the basics. How to breathe, socialise, date, dance, kiss, go to weddings, do Christmas, do *life* without alcohol. So here, we're going to cover that which I haven't told you about: years five, six and seven.

Once we're over three years sober, we're officially in long-term recovery, says popular opinion. The reason? A landmark eight-year study found that relapse rates plummet once we celebrate three years alcohol-free.

In the first year, 36 per cent sustain sobriety. It's a slippy-slidey time, and there's no shame in that, for the record. It took me five months of stop, start, stop, start, stop, to finally nail a Day One that stuck. Then, in year two, the success rate becomes 66 per cent. Great odds! After a three-year soberversary, we're looking at a magnificent 86 per cent staying sober.

Phenomenal; only a 14 per cent falter rate. But hang on, pipes up the negative-seeking drone inside me; that's not zero, is it? That's still 14 per cent. And the central theme of my last few years has been about that number, if I had to be a reductionist. About casting around for ways to feel as protected from it as humanly possible. Not living in fear, but being productive in protecting this rainforest from deforestation.

Early to mid-term recovery is an absolute blast, but also a terrifying tightrope, whereas from year four on, you've totally gotten used to not feeling like an extra from *Walking Dead* on a Saturday morning, so the gleam of that wears off. Making 9am yoga class feels less like a revelation, and more routine. 'So what?'

The congratulations for clocking up sober year after sober year, previously gobsmacked and awed, become bored. 'Oh, it's been six years?! Great!... *Looks at menu*. So, are we having starters or no?' It's your new normal. It's the new normal for everyone around you too. It's not a magnificent triumph any more. It's just how you live now.

Staying sober from year four on became, dare I say it, easy. But the less obvious yet more profound work began. I started finessing life skills that seemed like they were nothing to do with sobriety, yet they were *totally related*. I learned how to do things like say no (regularly), set boundaries (*hate* boundaries), ask for what I needed, preserve my energy for the parties I wanted to spend it on and learned how to open the chamber of shame (*the things I'd done*) in safe company. I'll be frank, much of this was less fun, but ultimately more transformative.

It was as if in years zero to four I'd learned how to dive to 18 metres, but from year four on, I started becoming a divemaster who could go to 30 metres. It was a bit darker down there at times, and the gear to get there was more awkward and advanced, but the experience was equally as exquisite.

I was already happy as a sober. Happy as a clam, happy as a camper, happy as Augustus Gloop in Charlie's Chocolate Factory. I had a brief spell of feeling bored, but that was soon torpedoed by a clever therapist who cleared his throat and said, 'Maybe you're just bored in general?' 'What do you mean?' I asked? 'Maybe you're just bored with your life right now, rather than bored with sobriety?' Hot damn, he was right. So, I went out and got a more interesting life. YouTube is your free friend, whether you want to learn to sea-swim or make a soufflé.

So I wasn't unhappy and I wasn't bored, but my challenge in long-term recovery was this. *How to finally feel safe.* Safe from myself, safe from others, safe from my memories, and last but definitely not least, safe from alcohol and the ultra-pressurised culture around it. That's what we're going to explore here. My first book was about finding the 'happy'. Here, we're going to plunge into the 'ever after'.

The sober revolution vs Big Alcohol

So, let's get up to speed. What's been happening in the past few years, on the drinking landscape? Well, first up, 2020 NHS data found that stereotypical perceptions of heavy drinkers are skewwhiff, given drinking is more common among the privileged who live in cushy areas. La-di-drinking-da. It's those with wine fridges (or even cellars), paddleboards, Farrow & Ball paint and fancy flavoured vodkas that are the lushiest boozehounds of all.

The same data re-confirmed that the biggest drinkers among us are Baby Boomers aged 55 to 64. Of that age bracket, two in ten women – and four in ten men – smash through more than 14 units a week on a regular basis. And no great wonder, given they grew up in the Babylonian, groovy, smoky and boozy, *Mad Men*-esque sixties.

Back then, some pregnant women in Ireland were prescribed half a Guinness a day for iron (true story: happened to my granny). The health messaging around alcohol has changed galactic amounts in the lifetime of Baby Boomers. Which probably makes it a bit bloody tricky to wrap their heads around. Or has created one hell of a dependence knot to unpick. A knot that could fox a sailor.

Nonetheless, there's also been a steady decline in binge – and regular – drinking overall. Fifty per cent of women and 35 per cent of men didn't have a drink in the past week. Yabbadabbadoo! Also, men drinking more than eight units in a session dropped to 19 per cent (this was 24 per cent 12 years ago). While women drinking more than six units in a sitting (that was just a *starter*, for

Drinking Me) dropped from 16 per cent to 12 per cent.

Millennials continue to swerve booze en masse. A 2019 survey found that a third of them planned to host a teetotal Christmas. Given Generation X and Boomers traditionally see the 25th as a day to drink from 10am (buck's fizz breakfast while opening presents!) through to midnight, this is mind-boggling. Almost half of the Millennials even said they'd drink tea or coffee, instead of lashings of wine, with their Christmas dinner. Show-offs. It's no surprise sales of no/low-alcohol beer are up 30 per cent since 2016.

And then – BOOM – national lockdowns 1.0 and 2.0 exploded, throwing all of our mental health not just off-track, but so far from the track, it could no longer even see the track. The pandemic concertina-pushed the nation's drinking at either end of the scale. A study by Alcohol Change UK found that while a fifth of Brits drank more (eep), a third drank less (yippee) and 6 per cent quit altogether (fucking A).

Big Alcohol's stealth marketing

In a fascinating contradiction, as the general public (not just the under 40s) increasingly teetotals, whether mostly or totally, the alcohol industry desperately floods socials with pro-drinking memes (because believe me, that's where these originate) saying things like, 'Holiday rules are airport rules: have a drink at 9am if you want to!' They're the equivalent of the spurned lover who packs their socials feed with flattering selfies, having just been dumped.

We need to get wise to this stealth marketing, this pro-bingeing content that is filtered into socials. If equivalent memes were released saying, 'I smoke because my kids are assholes', or, 'Keep calm and eat beef', we'd find them perplexing (and perhaps suspect tobacco/meat-industry inception), rather than lemming-like hitting 'share'.

Meanwhile, the booze-pushing guff, I mean *gift* industry has gone unregulated for donkey's years. But now, Watchdogs appear to be finally starting to stem the tidal wave of sparkly pink tat on the high street that endorses heavy drinking. In 2018, a goliath glass that could hold an entire bottle of wine was whipped off shelves.

In a landmark move in 2020, the Scottish Gin Society was slapped down by the ASA (Advertising Standards Authority) for suggesting gin was a healthier choice than a banana. Errr? In the same clean-up, the ASA also banned posts such as, 'Shut up liver, you're fine!', as well as a drawing of a stick man called Bill, accompanied by the caption, 'Bill has chosen to follow Ginuary, not Dry January. Bill knows January is a long month. Bill is smart. Be like Bill.' Ugh.

The pushback against Big Alcohol is finally mobilising, but for fuck's sake, given alcohol-specific deaths are still on the rise worldwide, it needs to *move faster*. I will tell you tales of tentacle-deep corruption between our governments + Big Alcohol later on that will have you squeaking with outrage. (There may also be a pattern enclosed for a dapper conspiracy-theorist tin-foil hat. Haven't decided yet.)

How's this book going to be different?

Betcha thought my previous books were gritty. Well, kiddos, we're about to get even grittier. I'm going to tell you tales of sexual indiscretions and infidelities, including why I'm (still) haunted by King Kong. Stories of drug-taking, the time I thought I'd killed a dog, the brush with Hackney Police, the lies I told romantic partners. I'm going to tell you things I've never told anyone, let alone published before.

Best of all, I've had the privilege of featuring 50+ voices in here that are not mine. We'll hear a sickie-chucking 'My gran died' story that is impossible to read without curling your toes and going 'eeeee'. We'll hear from the LGBTQIA community on why sobering up is much harder in a movement literally born in a bar. We'll hear from a mother who was told she'd ruined a four-year-old's birthday by not drinking. We'll hear about wine clanking under pushchairs and 3pm drinks in the park, about alcohol-curious teens and drinking to soothe post-natal depression.

Doctors have joined the confessional, telling us why they think their profession is three times more at risk of cirrhosis. Teentotallers will tell us how their twentysomething housemates are more supportive of their non-drinking than their parents. Men will share how zero-proof beer saved them from chest-beating, binary 'don't be a pussy' intoxicated masculinity.

We'll hear about the terrible twins – the tandem addiction of alcohol and cocaine – from those who are expert and those who have been there. There's a group-share about our most unexpected triggers, such as illness, PMT, summer, procrastination, phone calls, big-event sex and, oddly enough, productivity. And finally, women will share about being heavily pregnant, hounded by 'one won't hurt' social pressure. And about taking sips to avoid conflict while breastfeeding.

Much that I've merely brushed my fingers against previously now has room to grow and breathe. For instance, the bonkers rising trend for the wellness industry to push booze, previously a six-word mention, runs around in a full eight-page report. I've written a few sentences before about the astonishingly high link between a rough childhood and addiction: here, we'll explore that at length.

One thing will stay the same. Some in long-term sobriety get old-timer guru complex, where they stroke their beards or flick their hair and dispense wisdom as if it's an absolute. Definitely listen to all wisdom, but know this: we all make our own way, cherry-picking what works, and chucking what doesn't.

Me? I will never tell you that my way is The Way. All I have is lived experience and a geeky fascination for all things addiction- and sobriety-related. Given I am *no expert*, I call upon actual experts, constantly, and draw upon academic sources, persistently, to help me out in my quest.

The burning perennial questions

We'll also delve into some of the biggest, thorniest, juiciest, omnipresent questions. Does calling yourself an 'addict' or 'alcoholic' improve your chances? Is there any such thing as an addictive personality? Once an addict, always an addict?

These powder kegs, that regularly blow up comment boards from here to Timbuktu, will be explored with the help of my panel of exemplary experts. But as you'll see, even they disagree. Which illustrates that the only true 'fact' we can be sure of is this; there is very rarely a question for which there's a definitive yes/no, black/white answer. We can only posit opinions based on observations, or theories based on research, or beliefs based on what we've read.

In fact, that was one of the biggest things I learned, as a newly hatched sober. That black/white does not exist. I could finally see the infinite shades of grey. That many things I thought were 'fact' were actually just my opinions. That others were entitled to theirs. That I didn't have to try to wrestle their opinions to the floor and dominate them into tapping out. We could just both.... be. Co-exist. Politely nod to each other and leave each other alone. Rather than throw down on the mat.

I'll present what the experts think, and often what I think too. I'll also frequently showcase opinions and beliefs that contradict mine (as much as I would love to believe I know it all, it seems that I don't). And then: you decide.

You are an intelligent being entirely capable of coming to your own conclusions. I'll leave you to do the heavy lifting on deciding what *you* believe. Or possibly more pertinent: what version of reality helps you the most. If it soothes and benefits you, hold it tight with all your might. Don't let anyone take it from you, including me.

Ready? Let's go.

I hope you're excited, because I most certainly am.

A POSTCARD TO THE SOBER-CURIOUS

Dear sober-curious,

Welcome! At the risk of sounding creepy, *I can see you.* Here are some signs you're in the right place.

1. You feel mildly insulted by the prospect of one drink ('What's the point?!').

2. You find that alcohol suspends your anxiety, phew, but then re-animates it in an even grislier fashion the morning after, as if brought back from the dead via ill-advised sorcery.

3. Memories of drunken sexual encounters that make you shudder, even years later.

4. It's not unusual for you to have to go back to a bar or nightclub in order to pay off a monstrous tab you forgot to pay, or to ask them if they've found your bag/coat/wallet/laptop/passport/DJ decks (last one: for a friend).

5. Googling 'Am I an alcoholic?' on private mode at 1am.

6. Alcohol-induced rips in your memory. Once our blood alcohol goes over a certain amount, the hippocampus stops storing long-term memories, hence why we repeat

ourselves and forget entire hours/bars, but can still walk, talk and demand fried chicken.

7.   Two trips to the off-licence (liquor store) becomes standard because the amount you intend to drink, and the amount you actually drink, are always different.

8.   Or you've used one of those late-night 'dial 'n' drink' booze-delivery services because even though you'd had a skinful, you felt you could take on more at 2am. On a work night, no less.

9.   You refuse to confirm or deny reports that you have scrolled through pictures of you and your ex on Facebook, while crying into wine.

10. You have pushed a cork *into* a bottle of red wine rather than be forsaken by a crumbled cork. Or you've opened a bottle of booze with your teeth. Would you risk losing a tooth to drink some lemonade? I rest my case.

Back in my drinking days, I could say yes to *all* of the above. If you can say yes to many of these, you're in the right place. Come on in.

Catherine

THE TEMPLE OF BOON

I'm 15. I'm at a rave in Birmingham. 'Atomic Jam'. Or was it 'Spacehopper'? I'm not sure. I only know they all sound like raves held in space.

I'm here with my dreamy boyfriend, Matt, who is a small-time drug dealer. He's The One, so's you know. He and I sit on a bench and watch people whose inhibitions have flown from their bodies.

I've taken half of one of his pills, but nothing's happened. He's rolling. He rises, fist aloft, punching through the sky like a superhero as he comes up. 'Let's dance!' he cries, but I'm locked in my own skin, a prisoner of self-consciousness. I can barely stand up, let alone dance.

We haven't drunk a drop of alcohol, because the whole point here is to get high, not drunk. 'I haven't come up,' I whine. He bounces off and dances with another girl who is wearing a silver bikini and has pink hair. I wish I was that cosmic; she looks like a sexy alien.

A friend, Rich, comes and sits next to me. He's also a dealer. I choose the best people to hang out with.

'Where's Matt?' he asks. 'Dancing with her,' I say, miserably. 'My pill hasn't worked.' 'Where's his stash?' asks Rich. 'Inside my bra.' 'Take another half then, genius.' I go to the toilets, where two saucer-pupiled girls are stroking each other's faces as if their cheeks are made of velvet.

I take another half. Just as I swallow it down, the other half starts to move my jaw. Oh, shitttt. I am a baby ecstasy-taker, having only done it once before, and I'm not sure I can handle a full pill. Oh well. Fuck it. I paint another coat of glittery lip gloss across my face and smile, eyes dead, Joker-empty.

I care for my face and body as one might a treasured temple; buffing, polishing, painting. As for my insides? I plunder and ransack this temple for every boon, every bounty, every ill-gotten jewel of pleasure it can give me. I have no interest in the health of my internal self; only how the outside appears. The inside is a wreckage I plunder; the outside a tourist site.

I use cigarettes to daub dirty marks on my lungs, booze to push my way into hidden treasure chambers and, increasingly, I'm seeing that class A drugs can be archaeological diggers that unearth the subterranean stashes of pleasure that I heretofore couldn't access. They give me entry to underground boltholes crammed with pearls and overflowing chests. Bring. It. On.

I start dancing and can't stop; jerky and tireless like a wind-up toy. The bass owns me, as if I'm a bass-powered bunny. This hard house sounded vaguely like road works before; now it feels like angels beating drums. I hated this track – now I love it.

Rich's eyes light up when he sees me. 'BOOM!' he exclaims. He takes me around various rooms in this brokedown palace of a nightclub, using me as an advertisement for his product, pointing to my robotic toy dance and selling, selling, selling. I'm oblivious.

My boyfriend comes back to me from sexy-alien-silver-bikini. We are one. We go to hydrate, sit on bean bags and stroke each other's silk hair. Hair has never felt this good! Does hair always feel this good?

We say 'I love you', even though neither of us will mean it tomorrow. I go to the bathroom and see hot circles on my cheek, Pollyanna style, jjjjjh electric-shock hair, and a toothy smile that just won't quit, even when I try to physically close it. It pushes its way back open like an old-fashioned cash register. Ping!

Rubies tumble though my veins. Emeralds explode in my brain like fireworks. Previously crushed by my cares, I am now so unburdened of them that I feel I could actually fly.

The undulating crowd has found what it was seeking. That perfect togetherness, where the music twins with your soul and you feel you

belong, and every joke you make gets laughed at, and you feel as if
everyone likes you. We throw our hands in the air like we just don't
care, but the reality is: we all do. Way too much. Which is why we had
to get here artificially.

None of this is real. It's chemical. Ill-gotten bounty. I wasn't
supposed to access those underground boltholes. To dig them up. None
of us were. Because doing so comes with consequences.

It reveals too many riches, binges on them and leaves too little
for tomorrow – and the next day, and the next day. I am disrupting
the natural order of this pleasure temple. And I have angered the
guardians of it. There will be a ~~comeuppance~~ comedownance.

I spend the entire next week as a Temple of Doom. I drag myself
from home to school to home to school, a sad sack of flesh. I vow
never to take ecstasy again.

And all credit to me, I stick to it. Being the wind-up toy scared
me. Losing control scared me. My body felt like someone else's. But
it doesn't stop me trying other class As over the coming years, when
I want to plunder the forbidden pleasure caves.

I never pay for drugs, I never even obtain them, but if they're
there and convenient, I'll take them. Acid, cocaine, MDMA… but
mostly cocaine. Around 20 times over my lifetime.

Whyever not? I couldn't give two shits what the inside of the
temple looks like, as long as my body continues to do me favours
and as long as I'm withdrawing the jewels, and as long as the
external of the temple continues to draw approval.

My friends and I have seen these cosmically connected scenes on
Human Traffic, and *Trainspotting*, and even though the drug-taking
scenes are followed up with cautionary tales of addiction, we're all
seeking the magic one-ness anyhow. That star-aligning moment in
the night when everything feels like it's just right.

Each time we cheat our way there, the guardians punish us for our smash-grab.

Interestingly, I discover that they rumble more angrily about class As than the low dissent they give me about alcohol. I barely even feel hangovers, until I'm at university.

So, I concentrate on the alcohol. Alcohol brings lower boon, but less doom. It's my *thing*.

BURNING QUESTION: WHAT IS ADDICTION?

Throughout this book, I'll be dropping in 'burning questions' and letting you know what our panel of four experts think about them. These are the perennials that are discussed and debated over and over. (They most likely will continue to be, for hundreds of years still.)

What's fascinating to me is, you can ask a multitude of experts these very simple, oft-asked questions and you won't find two answers the exact same. It illustrates so very neatly that, when it comes to thinking about addiction, there is no one answer. There are many answers.

Our expert panel

- Dr Judith Grisel, Professor of Psychology and Neuroscience at Bucknell University. She's also the author of *Never Enough: the neuroscience and experience of addiction*.

- Dr Marc Lewis is a neuroscientist and retired professor of developmental psychology. He is the author of *Memoirs of an Addicted Brain and The Biology of Desire: why addiction is not a disease*.

- Dr Julia Lewis is a psychiatrist who has worked in the field of addiction for 15 years.

- Dr David Nutt is Professor of Neuropsychopharmacology at Imperial College, London and the author of *Drink? The New Science of Alcohol + Your Health*.

Dr Judith Grisel says: 'Addiction occurs when the debt becomes due. The debt we've created by borrowing our good feelings from the future. Some experts now say that it's a learning disorder. But it's more accurately described as a learning hyper ability. It's a perfect example of how terrific the brain is at learning, even though it's learned a self-destructive habit. We learn things more quickly when they're potent and meaningful. And to the brain, drugs like alcohol are inherently meaningful.'

Dr Marc Lewis says: 'Addiction is a very narrow category or set of activities or substances that seem to offer relief, pleasure or help for people who are generally struggling. Who are not finding that kind of relief in their social or cultural activities.'

Dr Julia Lewis says: 'A set of behaviours underpinned by elements of biology, psychology and social situation. Taking just the biology side, it's best described as abnormal learning. There are a very primal set of connections in the brain that drive us to repeat behaviours we need to survive: eat, sleep, mate, so on. Addiction hijacks that system, adding the drinking or gambling or drug-taking into the list of 'behaviours needed for survival'. Which means that when you don't do it, the internal disquiet and the upheaval in your reward system means you feel truly awful.'

Dr David Nutt says: 'Addiction is a behavioural state where you can't stop doing something, even though you no longer want to do it.'

Me: I'm chipping in just this once on a burning question, even though I'm no expert. Why? I get asked this question a lot.

For me, addiction is this: reaching for an external thing or person to change the way you feel. And it's a spectrum, of course, rather than something you can nail to the page. It's a continuum, not a black/white, yes/no binary.

The difference between addictive behaviour and non-addictive behaviour is really very simple. Once you start, you find it challenging to stop. Your best intentions get strapped to a rocket and blasted off into the ether.

Addictive behaviour around alcohol is thus. It doesn't matter if you only drink twice a week, or you only drink low-alcohol ale, or you always remember everything, or you never take your trousers off in public, or, or, or.

The dead giveaway is, you set out wanting to drink a certain number of alcoholic beverages, but the lion's share of the time, you drink more than that. You consistently set out on a night's drinking thinking, 'I am going to drink X' and instead you consistently drink Y. That's it. If you consistently drink more than you intend to, that is the red flag.

Think about it. Where else in life do you do that? I don't go out intending to have two soft drinks and then have four. I don't buy a whole cheesecake, intend to have one slice and then consistently, predictably eat all of it, despite trying, trying, trying to stop doing so (I realise many struggle with this, and my sympathies go out to them). Thus I do not have a dependence on cheesecake. Simple. Cheesecake is not my thing.

I do, however, frequently pick up my phone intending to look at it for ten minutes, and find that – whoosh – an hour has slipped by. Therefore, I am somewhat (not heavily, but kinda) addicted to my phone. Like most of us are.

Alcohol *was* my thing. My phone *is* my thing. And if alcohol is yours too, know this: there is nothing wrong with you. Only something wrong in the widespread notion that all of us should be able to 'take or leave' something wildly addictive. OK? OK.

Steps off glittery soapbox and drops mic

I: YEAR FIVE

YEAR FIVE: THE NEW MORAL NORMAL

In year five, I really started to relax – aaaahhhh – star-shaped into the knowledge that my life-savaging immoral antics were not going to return to prank me. They weren't going to burst back onto the screen, like a malevolent, mocking clown with a gun, that we haven't seen since Act One.

When I first dipped my toe into sober-land and started telling the truth about the most outrageously shameful things I'd done, I expected to be met with self-righteous preach. 'You did what?! You BAD drinker!'

I couldn't have been more wrong. If you tell a sober gang something you think puts you on a par with Attila the Hun, you can bet your bottom dollar that someone will chip in and go, 'You think that's bad?! Pull up a chair and hear what I did, sport!' Sobers are like the Jackanorys of hair-raising boozy stories.

Infidelity, stealing, wasting police time, calling in sick and driving over the limit are all astonishingly common offshoots of dependent drinking. Which means that sober land gets it. It's a safe space in which to shuffle off the coil of regret. To open the chamber of shame.

A magnet to a compass

Alcohol is to our moral compass what a magnet is to an actual compass. It banjaxes it. True North is no longer visible. But why is this? What's the science behind it?

'Ordinarily, questionable behaviour is held in check by your prefrontal cortex,' says neuroscientist Dr Grisel. 'The prefrontal cortex is like an overbearing parent. "Do this, don't do that! If you do that you'll look stupid! That's wrong, stop that!" Inhibitions and your moral compass come from the cortex,' she explains.

Only, when you're drinking, Dr Grisel says, this moral compass goes offline. 'The prefrontal cortex is the first part of the brain to go sleep. Which feels great, initially. You feel free. But it then leads to the bride crying in the bathroom on their wedding day, or the groom fist-fighting. Because, right now, they have fewer inhibitions. The "parent" is asleep.'

There's no longer a responsible adult in the room and thus bedlam ensues. Your brain is now not unlike an unchaperoned teen having a party ('Let's put our address on Facebook!').

We regress, essentially. 'The drinker has dropped down into the subcortical brain; the areas of motivation and emotion,' says Dr Grisel. 'They're in the limbic structures, where feelings and urges are processed. If they drop further beneath that, they're in the brain stem, which is comparable to the consciousness of a snake.'

Gosh. Comparable to a snake. I put this to Dr Grisel. 'So we devolve, over the course of a night's drinking?' She nods. 'Essentially, yes.'

Bring to mind the iconic illustration of us evolving from apes into upright homo sapiens, the one featuring five figures. Got it? Well, it's like we've rewound a step. No wonder our drunken priorities are primitive. We want to snog (rather than stay committed), fight (rather than nurture our friendships), dance (rather than get to bed early on a work night) or eat unidentified meat from a skewer (when we're veggie).

But alcohol doesn't do bad things, people do

In response to science such as this, we hear incarnations of, 'But alcohol doesn't behave badly, people do!' Which is reminiscent of, 'Guns don't kill people, people do.' And hell yeah, they have a point. There's still a person doing a bad thing. And that person is accountable for that bad thing.

However, the bad thing probably wouldn't occur without the conduit, the enabler, the catalyst – the gun or the booze. So this is not an argument that blows the need for gun control – or indeed alcohol awareness/policy reform – out of the water. It's much more nuanced than that.

Why do I think that immoral behaviour is sometimes alcohol-provoked? Here's a quirk; a flaw in the theory that the immoral act is 'the person', rather than the more complex interplay of 'the person + alcohol'. How come, when we stop drinking, many bad behaviours often evaporate – whoosh! Poof! Gone – for ever – without any effort whatsoever on our part? Doesn't that suggest that some immoral behaviours simply wouldn't have happened if we hadn't drunk? I believe so.

That doesn't mean, for the record, that I think a court of law shouldn't be able to throw the book at us for that immoral act. I'm not saying a 'drunk' plea should behave like an 'insanity' plea. Heck no. That would be chaos.

The genie in the bottle

Yet, it's official: alcohol is a drug that alters us. Our brains literally function differently. But our culture has a blind spot around this. A blind spot that we simply don't have around other drugs.

We know that every other drug alters us, inserts faux emotions and makes us behave out of character. We know to handle with caution. Cocaine made me feel silken and invincible, MDMA made me feel like I loved total strangers and, on acid, I gawked at an ornament smashing (I saw it in slow-mo) as if it was a gorgeous cosmic event. 'That's the most beautiful thing I've ever seen.' It wasn't, of course. The drug made me *feel* like it was.

With alcohol, we think it releases our core selves, like releasing a genie from a bottle. This just isn't accurate. *It is not true.* Your core self is who you are when you're sober. Of course it is. It's obvious, when you think about it. I bang on about this all the time, because it's incredibly important.

It's an almighty relief for those who get sober to discover that now that they're not getting twisted, their morals are no longer twisted either. To find that their behaviour has untangled from perverted to largely wholesome, just by virtue of putting a different thing in their glass.

Here are some of the ways my morals untwisted, without effort, purely as a result of quitting. You may relate.

1. I STOPPED CHEATING. 100 PER CENT

The chances of cheating when drunk are astronomical, when compared with cheating while sober. A 2017 study published in *The Journal of Sex Research* found that 70 per cent of cheaters give the main reason for their infidelity as: 'I was drunk and not thinking clearly.' So, seven in ten infidelities are enabled by alcohol.

Meanwhile, a 2016 study of over 800 university students discovered that drinking was a 'significant' predictor of cheating. 'Individuals who engaged in problem drinking were more likely to engage in sexual intercourse with someone other than their partner,' the study genteelly said.

No shit, Sherlock. I mean, we know this, don't we? But what is rarely talked about is this: how often the 'drink 'n' cheat' pattern is cured by one simple change. Quitting drinking. Bosh – cheating cured.

Before recovery, I thought my cheating was irrefutable proof I was a reprehensible, despicable, morally malfunctioning human being. I spent great swathes of time, forehead concertinaed, meditating on how I was going to stop my doggone no-good cheating ways. In fact, my cheating was the impetus for most of my failed runs at moderation. It was one of the things about my drinking that bothered me *the most*.

Desperately trying to cover up infidelities leads to a complex web of lies. We box ourselves in with lies. We need to remember them, in order to not lose our relationships. To avoid the tripwires that would sound the alarm. I often felt like a high-end burglar in a catsuit, staring at a criss-cross of scarlet lasers in between me and safety. I was going to have to backflip my way out of this.

Take the time I stayed late in the pub and kissed someone who wasn't my boyfriend. Instead of just telling my boyfriend I'd stayed late in the pub, and omitting the forbidden kiss, which would have been simplest, I inexplicably decided to tell him another story altogether. That I'd been to see the *King Kong* reboot, with my friend Ed.

'I've been dying to see that!' he exclaimed. 'Tell me all about it!' *Shiiitt.* I excused myself for an urgent loo break and Googled it on my BlackBerry (Millennials: I know you won't believe this, but they were all the rage then, OK?) to give him a potted plotline, before abruptly about-facing the subject.

I was terrified he would bring it up again, so I decided to go to the cinema, alone, to see *King Kong*. I needed my alibi to be watertight. Only, cinematic showings had now ceased. Fucksticks. I would have to wait for the DVD release! I read articles about it, but

I needed to *see it* to feel OK.

King Kong became a supersized emblem of my guilt. Any mention of King Kong, or anyone associated with the movie – Naomi Watts, Jack Black, Peter Jackson – now had the power to prick my scalp with beads of sweat. Giant monsters in general were now conversation starters I was phobic of – Godzilla, Bigfoot, even the Loch Ness monster or BFG. Because what if they set my boyfriend off again on *what I thought of the movie.*

Of course, it also set off a chain reaction of paranoia about Ed. Because if he saw Ed, and happened to mention it to Ed, then my cover would be blown to smithereens, and my boyfriend would dump me, and then I'd have to move out of our flat, and I'd probably lose my job, and end up properly homeless, and most likely then *just die.*

As you can see, I was catastrophizing this to the max. The mental gymnastics around blasted *King Kong* were exhausting. When I finally saw the damn thing, I sat there miserably, an unfaithful film swot.

Of course, my boyfriend never mentioned it again.

I thought the solution to the angst around my infidelities was thus: to locate the Atlantis of moderate drinking, go home at midnight, grow better morals; or beat myself up on a daily, hourly, minute-ly basis about my transgressions.

Turns out, the solution was elementary, my dear Watson. *Not drinking.* I thought my propensity for infidelity was an inbuilt character flaw, but it wasn't. In sobriety, fidelity comes as naturally as breathing.

'I thought you had a *cheating* problem, but not a drinking problem,' a friend said to me when I quit. Me too. But I was wrong, given the cheating was vanquished the moment I stopped drinking. With no mental effort on my part whatsoever. The prospect of cheating on a partner wouldn't even *occur* to me now, let alone manifest in an action.

I'm not telling you this to virtue signal. 'Get me, with my flawless fidelity!' *flicks dust off shoulder*. I'm telling you this because: if I could time-hop and tell the angst-ridden, self-lacerating 26-year-old me this, I would. And I honestly think she'd have quit drinking sooner as a result. So here I am, telling you too.

It may give you some hope, if you're still feeling lost. If King Kong's equivalent haunts you too. If you too are scared of the monsters under the bed.

2. I STOPPED SHOPLIFTING

I've written before about my having stolen alcohol. Not from shops, but from friends and family... as if that's any better. Twice, maybe three times, I have liberated a bottle from an overflowing wine fridge, telling myself they won't miss it, and I need it more than them. Innumerable times, I have siphoned other people's spirits, particularly housemates' vodka or gin.

I'll never forget having topped up a housemate's vodka with water, to hide my pilfering. However, he kept his vodka in the freezer, and now that the vodka was no longer pure vodka, the bottle promptly froze. He removed it from the freezer in front of me, going, 'What the Dickens...'

I've never written about my shoplifting, though, so let's get into that. Mostly, it was a teenage activity and is something a quarter of Brits admit to doing when they were a kid, said a 2020 YouGov survey. As teens we do tend to experiment with pushing the boundaries, just to see what we can get away with. But, boundary-pushing is even more prolific in boozehounds (see page 68 for some science on this). And we don't always grow out of it.

From the age of 14 to 17, a friend and I would slide a packet of cookies, or a sausage roll, into our school blazers. 'I know what you're doing!' the kindly corner shop owner would say, shaking his fist after us, but he would still let us come in the next day. (If that shop was still there, I would go and give him a £50 note and a sincere apology).

Then, I also did it as an adult too. Several times. Always when hungover, bizarrely. The illicit thrill of slipping a nail polish or a lipstick into my sleeve, and sauntering out, somehow pierced the wretchedness of my hangover.

As a sober, I never steal. I wouldn't dream of doing it, more's the point. I'm now very comfortable with following the rules. I even like colouring within the lines. Nowadays, I'm a fan of the lines.

Why the instant sea change from occasional shoplifter to law-observer? Well, we've already discussed how the prefrontal cortex goes offline when we're getting batfaced. But the PFC ('the parent' of the brain) also decreases in volume when that drinking is a regular and heavy event.

'Frontal lobes seem to be especially susceptible to volume loss following long-term chronic alcohol exposure,' said a 2014 study entitled 'The neurobiology of successful abstinence'. At the risk of over-simplifying an extremely complicated neuroscientific event: the prefrontal cortex loses synaptic density, or in laymen's terms; shrinks. Your moral compass/parent *shrinks*.

Thankfully, abstinence sees a snapback. It tends to regain that lost volume, the study says. 'The literature, while modest in size, suggests that abstinence is associated with improvement in prefrontal structure and function.'

In earthling language, our parent is back in the room. And it slaps our hand when we even *think* about putting a lipstick, or a packet of cookies, in our pocket.

3. I STOPPED BEING A DELINQUENT WHO WASTED POLICE TIME

Many of you will already know that I was arrested aged 27 in Brixton, a Bacchanalian part of South London, for being drunk and disorderly. I spent the night in the police station cell. In the morning, they returned my belongings. The only thing I had on my person? No keys, bag, phone. Merely a tiny, pink child's hairbrush, which I'd never seen before, and that had the audacity to be *glittery*.

But this particular story I'm going to tell you, this brush with the police, if anything makes me cringe more. Why? Because I wasn't completely blackout drunk when I behaved like an unspeakable brat.

While sober, I was a reliable, responsible and pleasant user of taxis. I would ask permission to drink a coffee in the cab, I would make polite small talk, I would admire the smell of their pine-tree air freshener, I wouldn't slam the door, I would give an extra pound even though I was always skint. Given my stepfather was (still is) a cabbie, I'd been raised to not be a tearaway in taxis.

But drunk, I was a cab driver's worst nightmare. I was a terror for hopping into taxis when I wasn't sure I had the money to pay for them. Most of the time, it was OK, given I would manage to hoodwink the cashpoint I stopped at into giving me a twenty (those standalone cashpoints in off-licences seemed less able to contact my bank for a 'Fuck no! Don't give her a penny!' result, so I favoured them. They charged £1.95 a pop, which I took as a bribe for them turning a blind eye).

Or if I was with others, they'd foot the bill, while silently glaring at me. Or there'd be a boyfriend on the other end of the phone who would agree to come into the street in their boxers, blurred with sleep, brandishing their wallet. (There'd always be a conversation in the morning about *never doing that again*.)

However, aged 26, there was one episode when all of my fare-dodging and cashpoint-whispering tactics fell foul. I was alone and had returned from two cashpoints empty-handed; even the dodgy one in 'Wine Not!'. My boyfriend, who I lived with, was (how-very-dare-he) unavailable at 1.26am on a Thursday morning. And so, my black cab driver decided to take me to a police station in Hackney. As he had every right to do, given I was unable to pay him for the service he had provided.

He was inside the police station, telling them all about the Nightmare Freeloader he had locked in the back of his Hackney Carriage. I cracked the manual window. Deep sighed. What a predicament. And then had an idea. I wriggled the window all the way down and managed to get my sequin mini-dress clad body through and out. FREEDOM!

I walked past the glass doors of the police station, side-glancing at the driver's gesticulating back, and weaved on up the street. Knowing better than to run, because only guilty people run, I beamed into the darkness, put my headphones in and started blasting Lily Allen, singing 'Fuck you! Fuck you very, very much'. I felt like a *gangster*.

Until, I sensed a presence beside me. A vehicle kerb-crawling me. I ignored it, until I heard 'Oi! We watched you crawl out of that window, love'.* I turned. To see: a police car, with two police officers inside. They took me back to the station. They were very friendly, considering.

Instead of charging me, they decided to allow me the privilege of seeing if my cohabiting boyfriend would pay for me. We turned up to my flat, where I eventually managed to outfox the dancing

---

* They may not have said 'Oi' or 'love' but my memory has filled in where the tone and exact words should be, with a Cockney stereotype of a copper.

keyhole and dominate it with the key (there were always liberal scratch marks around every keyhole where I lived).

They followed me in. The bedroom door was open and there my boyfriend was, stark bollock naked, spreadeagled, snoring. The police officers shielded their eyes from this too-much-info nudity. 'Ask him to put his clothes on before he comes to talk to us,' they said. They escorted my poor boyfriend to the cashpoint, where he withdrew £30 to pay my taxi bill.

In total, I probably wasted a good half hour of police time, and a half hour of the cab driver's time too, for whom time was money. The penalty should have been much worse. I wish they'd charged me, in retrospect. But they didn't. I don't have a record, but I should have.

It seems topsy-turvy that I should believe in consequences, while also championing radical compassion for addicted drinkers. But I do. Because consequences, as draconian and grim as they feel in the moment, often serve as convincers that propel that person from the darkness into the light.

4. I STOPPED CHUCKING SICKIES*

My nickname, at one workplace, was the very fetching 'Sick Note'. Not only did I lie about endless dodgy prawn curries, fake the raspy voice of a flu, faux a limp for an entire week (Keyser Söze, *Usual Suspects,* eat your heart out) and memorise the symptoms of migraines from Wikipedia, I even lied about fake funerals too. *I know.*

I killed off one grandpa who was already dead. A few times, in fact. I told myself that it was OK because he was already deceased.

---

* International readers: a 'sickie' is British slang for being absent from work for being 'ill', when you're actually hungover.

I moved the date of an aunt's funeral, in order to skip a day at my Saturday job and go see *The Rocky Horror Picture Show* with my boyfriend. 'Why is that woman staring at us?' I said to him, gesturing to a lady in liberal stage make-up, a red wig and a silver top hat. Turns out it was my boss.

Hangovers are actually the top reason we phone in sick, said a report from PwC. It sounds like the absolute height of selfishness, chucking a sickie, but often a severe hangover means waking into a scary predicament. And a physicality that would not be able to withstand work.

Shaking hands, a pounding head, a roiling stomach; we don't know if we can manage to pull off an Academy-Award-winning performance of a normal employee today, so we call in sick. We may have even spent all of our money and not have the funds for a travelcard; it's happened to me. Or we may have even woken up in a different city.

As a sober? All of this stops. And so sickies become totally unnecessary. It's a stunning relief.

The Chamber of Shame

One of the most common questions I'm asked is: 'What do I do with all of this shame? This guilt that I'm left holding, now I've stopped drowning it in booze?' My heart jumps out of my body and goes out to each and every person who asks me this. Because I know precisely how that feels. It's one of the reasons we tried to stay drunk, in the first place. To ignore the existence of the Chamber of Shame.

It's stating the bleedin' obvious, but one of the most effective ways to put a pin in shame, to deflate the guilt, is to make amends to the person whatever-episode hurt. I have sent numerous messages, written in cards and delivered heartfelt apologies to those I have hurt with my thoughtless drunk/hungover/generally narcissistic behaviour.

'I'm sorry that you recommended me for that job – and then I couldn't be arsed to do it properly,' for instance. Or to someone I had three dates with once-upon-a-time – 'I'm sorry you planned a lovely weekend for us and I showed up spangled, having drunk a bottle of wine on the train, and proceeded to shout at you over a lovely dinner you'd toiled over.'

Many people won't respond. The latter didn't. He read it, ignored it, blocked me. That's A-OK. That's his right. The very act of making the amend means we've done our bit.

But what if the person doesn't know about what you did to them? The rule of thumb goes that, if making amends would involve revealing something that would hurt that person *more* than the apology would soothe them, then you should probably keep it zippered. In this instance, you can make what AAers call 'living amends'. This means you just make up for your twonkish behaviour day by day, year by year, by being a lot less of a twonk.

Something that's constantly forgotten is this. Technically, amends should extend to yourself too. Because much of your behaviour hurt *you* more than anyone else. You could even write a letter to your body and mind, saying something along the lines of: 'I'm sorry that I put you in danger; I'm sorry I poured litres of a neurotoxin into you; I'm sorry I starved you of sleep and nutritious food. I promise to never treat you so carelessly again.'

The unpack of the chamber

For the shame echoes that you can't amend away – that echo, feel, cringe, repeat, in your Chamber of Shame – here's what most people in recovery do. They unlock the chamber and do a long, arduous inventory of that which they have stowed away diligently and deliberately. They unpack. In the company of another sober person, usually, or alternatively, a professional counsellor.

In AA, they call this a Step 5: 'Admitted to God, to ourselves and to another human being the exact nature of our wrongs.' It's usually done with a trusted sponsor, who is bound by the AA pact that you sometimes hear chanted in meetings, 'What you see here, what you say here, what you hear here, let it stay here.' I can't comment on what it's like to do a Step 5 in AA, but I've been told by friends who love the program that I've motored through many of the steps without even realising it.

Being ready to do my interpretation of a Step 5, took me a l-o-n-g time. I'd cracked the door and unpacked some of it, for sure, but I was over four years sober when I unpacked *the whole thing*.

Many think a Step 5 is best done quickly; they think you need to open, stare down and exorcise the Chamber in order to stay sober. For me, it was the opposite. I needed time with Cath 2.0, before I could fully forgive Cath 1.0. I needed that respite. Things had been dark for so very long.

So, come my fifth year, I itemised my worst wrongs on a sunshine-drenched day, with one of my best sober friends, Jen, while wearing a bikini with tangerine slices on it. It felt like the day was so bright, I could stand to open into the darkness. I removed every object of shame, of guilt, of self-loathing, and showed it to her. Every time I showed her one of mine, she showed me one of hers.

I only told Jen because I trust her implicitly and she was sharing alongside me. The joint nature of it felt safer. We now both know so much about each other that we could easily cut letters out of magazines and send a blackmail note. *I know what you did in the summer of '99. Pay up or else!* Not that we ever will.

For that very reason, though, I would be exceptionally careful about who you choose when you unlock the Chamber of Shame. The only other people I have opened the contents in the presence of, have been trained therapists who are bound by confidentiality.

The truth about shame is that time is the great healer. There's no substitute for it. The more you show yourself – and others – that you are now a different human, the more the shame recedes. You evolve into the person you were meant to become all along, before addiction threw you off course. The longer time ticks its inexorable way on, the more you forgive yourself. You no longer feel haunted by your past mistakes; or hunted by the prospect of their reveal.

Your behaviour now matches your morals. You begin to exhale, fully. To feel safe in your own skin. To trust that this is how it is now. And you realise – *this is me.* That was *not me.*

> *'I have already lost touch with a couple of people*
> *I used to be.'*
>
> Joan Didion

ACCIDENTAL DRINK-DRIVING

Thankfully, I never drove drunk, simply because I never *drove*. But I know that if I had started driving in those years, I would have driven over the limit. For certain. So, there's zero judgement loaded into what I'm about to say.

Many binge drinkers accidentally drink-drive in the morning, with alcohol still jiving through their system like John Travolta, utterly oblivious that they would fail a breathalyser.

The enormously useful Morning After Calculator app shows how long we take to metabolise alcohol. It may be eye-opening to find out that:

- If you drink one bottle of wine (or 10 units) and stop at midnight, you can't drive until 11am the next morning.

- If you drink two bottles of wine (or 20 units) and retire at midnight, you're not OK to drive until 9pm the next evening.

- Thus, it's safe to assume (even though the app won't allow us to input half bottles of wine), that if you put away 1.5 bottles of wine (or 15 units) and stop at midnight, you shouldn't drive until 4pm.

I know. Given my usual intake in the last few years of my drinking was minimum a bottle, usually a bottle-and-a-half, it's a good blinkin' job I didn't have a driving licence.

SICKIE GROUP-SHARE

I asked a bunch of readers to tell me about the juggernaut-proportioned lies they've told in order to wriggle out of work. The ones that still fly through their conscience like a zeppelin, even many years on.

The most commonly cited bum-clenchers of the 53 I received were: the faking of deaths of relatives (both those already dead and those still alive). Each of these came with a huge serving of lingering guilt. So if you've faked a death/funeral too, know this: you're not an evil outlier. Your lie is actually pretty unoriginal. Just be glad we don't have to do that shite any more.

Here's a selection of the best stories I received.

'Before cellphones, I drove for two hours to a different city and used a roadside pay phone there to call my boss, saying my car had broken down. Given it had a different telephone area code, I thought it would be more believable. I then found the closest bar and got drunk all over again.'

Chris

'I was so hungover at work that I wanted to lie down and disappear. I went into the stationery cupboard and lay down on the floor, with a box next to my head. A friend found me. I said I must have been knocked out by the box falling off a shelf. The stationery cupboard probably stank of alcohol, but I got sent home nonetheless.'

Avery

'I said I was locked in my own flat. That I'd lost my keys the previous day and my flatmate had left for work and bolted the door. I was horrified when a colleague said his dad was a locksmith and he'd send him round!'

Farrah

'My go-to was always pink eye (conjunctivitis). It was perfect because a person with pink eye is basically akin to a leper; no one wants you anywhere near them. Plus it's good for two days. That's two days for you to get over your ungodly hangover, and if you turn up on the third day looking a bit squinty, people assume it's just a symptom.'

Audrey

'I said I needed to go to hospital having slipped on ice outside my house and hurt my wrist. I even went in the next day wearing a fake bandage!'

India

'My friends and I had a script for calling in sick if we had a male manager. We would always say "endometriosis" and talk at length about the lining of our uterus. It covered you for one bender every month.'

Willow

'Towards the end of my drinking, I emailed my boss to say my nana had died and I had to go home and help my mum with the funeral. People in work were so kind to me. I nearly slipped up a couple of times, mentioning I needed to send a Christmas card to her. And then quickly correcting myself, saying, "sometimes I forget she isn't around any more." God, it was awful. I've never told anyone, until now. Thankfully Nana is still alive and well, seven years after I told that horrendous lie.'

Grace

'After getting blackout drunk with a group from work (including my boss and some of my employees) there was no way I was making it in. I concocted this elaborate eye injury excuse and to really sell the point, I wore an eye patch for a whole three days. One of those huge, adhesive, maxi-pad-esque ones.'

Amaira

'In a moment of blind panic after a gin binge session, I told work that my nan had passed away. They sent flowers to my parent's home address. My parents were away at the time, so my nan went down to pick them up after a neighbour rang her. Thankfully she didn't read the note inside sending me condolences for her passing! I stopped drinking a few months later.'

Charlotte*

---

* All names have been changed. A colossal thank you to my Instagram followers who contributed. Over 50 of my readers are quoted in this book; in all cases pseudonyms have been used (see pages 53–6, 84–6, 115–20, 151–3, 158–61, 167–8, 212–17, 228–9). Without their candour, wit and wisdom, these sections would not have been possible.

STONE COLD VS SUNSHINE WARM OCEAN-GOING

STONE COLD DRUNK OCEAN-GOING

JULY 2011

'This is like something out of a rum advert,' I think satisfyingly, as myself and six friends recline on the deck of a catamaran. Reggae mingles with the rush of the waves as the prow of the Merry Barracuda *cuts through them.*

I'm in the Caribbean. Not ordinarily my holiday destination of financial scope but, due to a jammy turn of the wheel of chance, I have ridden on somebody's coat-tails here. It makes a change from my usual holiday haunts of Ayia Napa, or Zante, or somesuch budget holiday in a hotel that almost certainly has bedbugs.

My destinations are usually volcanic and stripped of green, but I don't give a damn; my pilgrimage is all about the neon-lit strip of bars with cheap drinks and fast men. And the sun, of course, which I bake myself under in the hope it will make me more attractive. I feel monstrous most of the time, apart from when I drink, when I feel silken and sexy.

I chase the holiday scenes I see in alcohol adverts, wanting to become the laughing surfer who spears her board in the sand and hops into a hammock with a cold one. Or the badass who takes a swig from a bottle before busting out a perfect-10 dive from a rocky outcrop, emboldened by liquid courage. The toned beach bombshell who lounges and sips from an umbrella-sheltered cocktail, never getting sand in her unmentionables.

But I never get there. I never seem to be able to make it happen.

I always have to take it too far; I go too hard, too fast, and my repeated moderation failures now spin me into frequent self-loathing. 'Why can't you become her, stupid, stupid, stupid?' my head heckles me.

What isn't televised is the secret hell of a holiday hangover. Which, for all I know, the others feel too, but none of us will talk about it. If we do confess to how diabolical we feel, then we know what the penalty is; to spend a night not drinking. So we struggle on, locked on our private hangover islands.

Everyone was up late last night and drinking hard, so it's likely that I'm not alone in my hangover on this ocean-going vessel. At 3am, when the others made their escape to bed, I managed to catch the toe of someone trying to flee, like a mouse by its tail.

I pulled her back with me and kept her until the bitter end of 5am. 'Don't be so BORING, we're on holiday!' Once I'd pounded my fill – eight beers and 15 menthol cigarettes – I released her from the hostage situation.

I eye my captive from last night. She snoozes on the deck, hat tipped over her face, hand curled around a two-litre bottle of water that she's nearly finished. H20? Really? H20 cannot possibly cure this hangdog hell; only the hair of the dog (that bit me) can. When I'm hungover like this I feel wired, rather than tired. How can she sleep?

My eyes are shrunken and shot through with bloody forked-lightning, but they're hidden behind knock-off market-stall aviators. The anxiety roils in rhythm with the ocean, building until I could scream. When I try to smile, all I can muster is a rictus grimace. The tremble in my hands feels like fizzy electric shocks, as if my body is short-circuiting.

'Reef!' calls the catamaran captain, joyously. My friends squeal and rush for the snorkels, including my hostage, lowering themselves into the spearminty water. They point their bodies towards the reef further inland, fins childishly flip-flopping.

Really. Must I? I just want to lie here and recover. I don't tend to bother snorkelling, given I am always much more interested in the caipirinhas than the coral, and chasing the local men rather than the local clownfish, but OK, if I must.

I descend into the unknown. Fucksticks. My anxiety was an eight, and now it's nudging a nine, as I tip my nauseous body horizontal in the water and pretend that I'm enjoying this ordeal. I'm well behind the others.

A large dark shape swims beneath me, as I leave the boat's safety. I surface, rip my mask off and ask the skipper, 'What the fuck was that?'. I address him accusatorily, as if he should have purged the Caribbean of scary shapes before I lowered myself into it. 'Probably tuna,' he says, shrugging, refusing to indulge my brattish strop.

'What if it's a shark?!' I say, now flailing in the water.

He shrugs again. 'Reef shark. Peaceful.'

I flounder my way back onto the boat, clown-footing my way up the ladder in my inelegant fins, which only serves to make me angrier. Nothing about this feels like a rum advert now! Given I live on the precipice of panic at the best of times, one unpredictable underwater shadow is enough to plunge me into the inkiest of depths. I hate the not knowing.

I tear the fins off, stomp downstairs to get a stubby beer from the fridge (why are these so fricking small?! Three mouthfuls and done) and sit on the deck, sulking, a shipwreck of a person.

I take another. And another. I drink three before they're back from their hour-long snorkel. The alcohol muffles the scream building inside me. It used to do so in a comforting way. But now it's more like a hand clamped over my scream, until I stop struggling. Until I'm limp.

SUNSHINE WARM SOBER
OCEAN-GOING

FEBRUARY 2020

My sober sister Laurie and I are in Thailand. We stretch out across the top deck of a boat, a boat filled with other boisterous snorkellers. There's a rainbow-painted slide that goes directly from the top deck into the sea, but even the Gen Zs with swagger, who are trying to one-up each other with their tinny phone music, find it too intimidating to actually use. People cannonball, swan-dive or accidentally belly-flop into the ocean.

We've been treated to rare sightings of unbleached coral, vivid as fistfuls of amethysts; giant clams that will snap if you touch them; scrappy triggerfish that will charge like a bull and bop you on the mask if you get too close; dreamlike jellyfish that look like they're ballet dancing to a soundtrack of opera.

The last stop on the snorkelling tour is Shark Bay. I'm now a qualified scuba diver who has seen reef sharks in the wild a few times, so I know not to listen to the 'dun dun, dun dun, dundundundunDUNDUN' Jaws music that builds in my head when I think about sharks.

You're much more likely to get bitten by a dog. Once you see an actual shark chasing a cuttlefish and not giving a flying fuck about you, you realise that most shark phobias are based on pure propaganda, courtesy of Hollywood. Very similar to getting-sober phobia, incidentally. Laurie isn't remotely scared of reef sharks either, so we swim to a part of the bay where there are the fewest people, to up our chances of shark-spotting.

When the first shark glides past, poetic muscle in motion, we burble with joy into our masks. Over the next hour, we see two, three, four black- and white-tip reef sharks. Or maybe the same ones over and over, who knows?

We're just about to head back to the boat when a fifth reef shark, a white-tip, emerges from the shadows. Six foot of shark. Unlike the others, who only stick around for a couple of seconds in sight before flicking their tails and heading in a different direction, he laps us.

He's on his second, closer lap when we start getting nervous. Laurie draws a lapping motion in the water. We know being circled by a curious shark is not ideal. That's the kind of scenario that leads to an exploratory charge and butt, or maybe even a nibble. But what can we do?

Then I remember there is something we can do. In PADI training, they teach that if you can't get beneath an inquisitive, circling shark (sharks invariably attack from beneath) given the water's too shallow (here on this reef, it is) then your best bet is this. Turn, face the shark and make yourself look as big as possible. Thrashing away in a panicked swim is the worst thing you can do.

So, I face the shark, flip myself upright and make myself into a human star. (I know, what a hero. In case you didn't get that subtle subtext.) But the reality is, this white-tip reef chap is practically harmless; only five recorded bites ever have occurred.

I still feel like a star-shaped hero, though. And, as promised by my divemaster teachers, the shark does one. Swims off immediately. It's just a rule of the wild; bigger wins. And I've just turned myself from a relatively small, long, thin thing into a bigger five-pronged thing.

We swim back to the boat sharpish, granted, but boy, do we feel powerful in that moment. We owned what power we could while also knowing that we could no more control the shark's response than you can turn off a tornado, or snip the moon's pull on the tides. Power – let go. Do what you can – let go. Be brave – let go.

We can control very little. But simultaneously, we are often more powerful than we think we are. And what gives us that power? Knowledge. Knowing as much as we can about the thing we're getting into the water with.

PLEASE DON'T SELL ME GIN DURING SPIN

INT. UNNAMED SPINNING STUDIO. LONDON.

A neon-lit billboard hangs above the spinning studio door. 'Detox, retox, repeat!' it announces.

I inelegantly clip-clop on my cleated shoes towards the bike, like I'm walking on ice skates. Most of the other spinners have the common sense to put the shoes on once they're actually on the bike. I'm not one of them.

I can't clip into the pedal thingummies. The instructor shows me how to do it.

I still can't clip in.

The instructor comes over to me and tells me, in a s-l-o-w 'talking to a dumbass' voice, how to do it.

I still can't clip in.

The instructor literally grabs my feet and clips them in.

It's a dignified start.

The lights are low, the mood is primal, and once the music kicks in, it's club-level loud. The instructor does a twirl and hops onto the bike, like a star bursting onto a stage.

A HALF HOUR LATER
The instructor: 'Push it, push it, push it. Imagine there's a bottle of gin at the top of this hill, team!'

She thrusts her fist into the air, like a spinning revolutionary. The crowd whoops, albeit in a half-awkward, John Cleese-esque, British way.

TEN MINUTES LATER

The instructor: 'And right after this class, you can have a free prosecco at our bar! It's free prosecco Fridays!'

The glistening, panting spinners whoop for real this time.

TEN MINUTES LATER

The instructor: 'Detox, retox, repeat, gang! Think of those cocktails you're earning! We work our asses off so that we can reap the reward!'

People beam into the darkness. Detox, retox, repeat!

After class, half of the studio goes straight to the bar (it also sells smoothies, FYI, but those were not mentioned) for a dehydrating prosecco. The other half rehydrates via the water fountain instead.

***

How many would have gone to the bar, I wonder, if alcohol hadn't been mentioned three times during our afternoon session? Probably zilch. The power of suggestion is a tug rope that takes us to the bar. Marketing is a wily sprite that dances in your mind long after the thing has been mentioned. Like Tinker Bell pirouetting, holding a branded bottle.

Gym with a side of vin

The wellness industry + alcohol wasn't *a thing* until recently. Otherwise, believe me, I would have taken a swing at it.

But now it is. And here's my theory around how this unfolded. Back in 2018, I would say we reached the zenith of alcohol-enabling memes. BOOM: they were everywhere. Drinkers love them, and they share, share, shared, just as I used to make notes of enabling quotes from famous people. (One of my favourites was 'Alcohol is like Photoshop for real life' – Will Ferrell.) We are big drinkers, and things that make us feel better about our big drinking *sell*.

The alcohol memes sensation made it even more clear to profiteers that an alcohol-enabling slogan was a crowd-pleaser. And so booze started infiltrating markets in which it has no place. Yoga studios started sending out teasers entitled 'Do you love gin… sorry, yin?' Click, clickety click, went their mailing lists. Spinning studios, like mine, started offering alcohol at their smoothie bars and finding their profit margins fattened. On it grew.

Finishers of obstacle courses such as Tough Mudder were inexplicably given a free beer at the end. Makes total sense! That's just what your body needs after an arduous sporting event, sure thing! If you don't drink, you don't get anything free, as far as I can tell from the Tough Mudder website. Why? It's not truly a perk. It's all about your wealth (marketing to hundreds of tired, muddy, impressionable new customers) and zero to do with your health.

Alcohol made its way onto sportswear and sports gear. Enter a Seventies style 'I was told there'd be wine' gym bag. 'Gym first, gin later' tops. 'No pain, no champagne' sweatshirts. Even a pink 'powered by prosecco' sports bottle. All of the above are real products, by high-end sportswear brands – not sweatshop tat – many of which you can still buy now. Whoosh! went the profits. The sports-brand bigwigs rolled around in beds full o' money, cackling.*

And so alcohol + sports was a hit. Ergo, some studios took this batshit gimmick and supersized it; by beginning to serve alcohol not just after, but *during their classes*. Right now, right here, where I'm writing to you from (late 2020), I can book a 'Yin yoga workshop & gin distillery experience'. Or 'Pinot Pilates' whose class motto is 'Inhale. Exhale. Sip. Repeat.' Or I can 'beGIN my

---

* Legal disclaimer: I have no actual evidence of this, sadly.

weekend' with the spin and gin. It's absolutely wackadoodle. Even when I was an addicted drinker, I would have found the presence of red wine during a Pilates class gonzo.

'When the ridiculousness of beer yoga *et al* started happening, Yoga Alliance sent an email to all members saying your insurance won't be valid if students are drinking in class,' says Eleanor, a yoga teacher. And so, studios and gyms started offering it afterwards instead. 'It's a marketing tool to pull in the people that normally wouldn't exercise,' says Olivia, a personal trainer. 'But it means people come in for the wrong reasons. For weightlifting and prosecco afterward.'

Olivia thinks that many of those who train, or run gyms and studios, are on the addictive spectrum themselves. 'Trainers are some of the biggest drinkers you can find. Many look influencer-fit and shredded, but are actually taking steroids or growth hormones, and then over-training and over-drinking.'

She thinks the stress of the industry drives this excess. 'It's over-subscribed and under-supported.' And in such a cutthroat, competitive environment, she says that 'likes' are king. 'The fact is that the 'detox then retox' style posts get a lot of likes. It's seen as a "sexy" lifestyle message, while sobriety isn't. I'm stronger, happier and healthier now I'm sober, but I don't see that reflected back at me in the fitness messaging.'

Of course, alcohol may be a new entry to the traditionally female-favoured sports like yoga and Pilates (at the risk of being horribly binary and reductionist, forgive me), but booze has been present in more stereotypically macho fitness (ditto, binary buzzer) for decades. Rugby and football are famously boozy, while even the players of darts and snooker are often lashed during the tournaments.

Snooker champion Ronnie O'Sullivan regularly played and

drank, before hitting rehab, which he called 'probably the best thing I've ever done'. Darts legend Andy Fordham asserted people never saw him sober and said he drank 24 beers before winning the World Championship. He's been teetotal since 2007.

The most insidious impact of alcohol + sports is that it gives booze a health glow it doesn't deserve. In a doctor's surgery today, I saw an NHS poster that said 'Alcohol is the second biggest risk factor for cancer, after smoking. How does that make you feel?' underneath a very sad-looking bulldog.

But then I walked past a muscle vest in a high-street window saying 'Strong men need strong drinks'. Later, in a gift shop, I saw a sports water bottle saying 'Vodka is vegan'. Back when I was a dependent drinker, this subliminal 'work out hard, drink hard' messaging would have allowed me to forget about the haunting bulldog. It's confirmation bias – we Velcro to that which supports our beliefs. And allow the other messaging to fall out the trapdoor marked 'inconvenient truths'.

Alcohol sports sponsorship

Then there's the multi-billion pound business of alcohol brands sponsoring sporting events. Take these two morally irreconcilable exhibits.

Exhibit A: In 2019, a study by three universities revealed that a bottle of wine a week is comparable to the cancer risk caused by puffing ten cigarettes for women, and five cigarettes for men. Alcohol and cigarettes are officially in the same carcinogenic classification.

Exhibit B: Jacob's Creek wine is a sponsor of the US Open Tennis Championships. In the UK, Lanson champagne sponsors Wimbledon.

When you add those two facts together, exhibit B becomes somewhat disturbing, does it not? That alcohol brands continue to be allowed to sponsor sporting events globally, and thus enjoy the rubbed-off gleam of fitness and sporting prowess. Tobacco sponsorship of sports was banned in 2003. And yet there's no great difference whatsoever between cigarette brands and alcohol titans sponsoring such tournaments.

Over a decade ago, the BMA (British Medical Association) and NICE (National Institute for Health and Clinical Excellence) called for an outright ban of alcohol brands being allowed to sponsor sports. In 2014, 36 health leaders wrote a letter to the *Guardian* calling for a ban too, saying that alcohol–sports advertising has become 'as commonplace as advertising for cereal or soap powder'.

The letter bemoaned the fact that children see their sporting heroes wearing shirts emblazoned with alcohol brands, and pointed out research that shows early exposure to alcohol advertising leads to earlier – and harder – drinking in youngsters. It added, 'Shouldn't our national sports be inspiring our children to lead healthy and positive lifestyles? It would be considered outrageous if high-profile teams like Everton or Celtic were to become brand ambassadors for tobacco, and so why is it acceptable for alcohol?'

Nothing happened. Absolutely zip. Meanwhile, other countries have wised up. Places such as France, Ukraine and Norway have outlawed such poppycock, while countries like Italy have severely restricted it. Why haven't we? It's confounding.

It's not like the money won't pour in from elsewhere. When Australia banned tobacco companies from sponsoring sports, sponsorship revenue actually *increased* nationally by 45 per cent. An article that appeared in the British Medical Journal revealed that, 'A UK simulation of a ban on alcohol and gambling sponsorship estimated that 84% of lost revenues would be replaced immediately by other sponsors.'

Unfortunately money opens a lot of doors, even if that money would promptly come in from elsewhere. FIFA's longstanding relationship with Budweiser saw Russia compromise its morals. Russia introduced a total ban on all alcohol advertising in 2012, in order to try and reverse rocketing rates of alcohol addiction. But then, Russia won the hosting of the World Cup in 2018. And it decided to temporarily reverse that decision. During the matches, the Budweiser logo was very much omnipresent on Russian soil, presumably because FIFA insisted upon it. Russia's morals 0, FIFA and Budweiser 1.

There are those who refuse to take the bait. The SWF (Scottish Women's Football) has promised never to accept sponsorship from alcohol companies. While teetotal and Muslim Egyptian goalkeeper Mohamed El-Shenawy refused to accept a 'Man of the Match' award emblazoned with the Budweiser logo, despite it being the first time an Egyptian player had won the award in the World Cup.

These small protests are a call for bigger change. It's high time that we started to object to an undeniably health-eroding drug being associated with health-boosting activities. Much like any implicit bias, this relies on us all calling it out, whether on a grass-roots level at our local yoga studio that has started serving wine after (or during!) classes on a Saturday, or boycotting sports brands that push beer on their muscle vests.

Alcohol + sports have no place together, just as tobacco + sport don't. 'Detox, rehydrate, repeat' may not have the same ring to it, but I'm chanting it in my head during my spin nonetheless. And I'll punch the air like a slightly awkward Brit any time; you don't need to offer me gin.

REAL SLOGANS
ON REAL SPORTSWEAR

- On your marks, get set, prosecco!

- Fitshaced*

- I like to rum

- Let's get fizzical

- Gin bunny

- Does running out of wine count as cardio?

- On a dancer's vest:
  'Trust me, you can dance.'
  Vodka

---

* To be fair, this play on 'shitfaced' did make me snicker.

THE ADJACENT 'FUCK IT' BUTTONS OF DRINKING & DEBT

In year five, I finally got out of debt. After having spent my entire adult life with minus-zero money, I finally clawed my way up to zero-plus. I heaved myself out of fire-alarm 'lies awake in bed' red, into the serene soporific black.* I never would have had the wherewithal to do this unless: sobriety.

Why? The 'fuck it' button of 'have another drink' lives right next door to the 'fuck it' button of 'spending money we don't have'.

It's very Captain Obvious of me to point out that big drinking leads to big debt. Of course it does. It's expensive. But what isn't often discussed is this – once you have that debt swinging over your head like a guillotine, it provokes you to drink *more*.

A 2013 meta-analysis of the health impact of debt found five studies that showed something startling. Those with debt were 2.68 times more likely to exhibit AUD (alcohol use disorder). It's impossible to know what came first, of course – the debt or the drinking – but we can safely say that debt is kindling for disordered drinking.

The more freaked out we are by our debt, the more likely we are to throw our best-laid plans into the air like confetti and dive to double-press both the 'drinking' and 'debt' buttons. Which looks like this:

Fuck it, I'll sort that bill next week, let's go and get clattered instead: **gets a late payment charge.**

---

* Farrow & Ball, I am available for paint-name brainstorming.

Fuck it, I'll miss the last bus home in order to have another drink: **needs to pay for a £30 taxi**.

Fuck it, I'll park here because I slept in and am too late to find a legitimate space: **gets a ticket**.

Fuck it, I'll skip my HIIT class because I can barely lift a pen, let alone a dumbbell: **gets a late-cancellation charge**.

Fuck it, I'll whack it on the credit card because I think *this thing* will ease my hangover: **is charged eye-watering interest**.

Once, I was in Rome with my first credit card in my 19-year-old paw. Said credit card came automatically with my student account, as did the overdraft; starter water wings for a lifetime of swimming in debt. I was hungover and decided that buying £150's worth of underwear would be the perfect cornflower-lace, peony-silk panacea. Yes! That is the answer. I will spend my way out of this profound existential dread!

Only, because I was in the mindset of living in today, and letting tomorrow go hang, I took about three years to pay it off via teeny tiny bare minimum payments, and thus £150 of underwear cost me, oh, around £600.

Why do we behave this way? It comes back to the prefrontal cortex again. Remember? The 'parent' of the brain? 'There's good evidence that the prefrontal cortex is less active in those in active addiction,' says Dr Judith Grisel. 'Which means that short-term pleasure has more meaning than long-term punishment. There's less cortical control at work; you're more driven by compulsive habit.'

The alcohol, the partying, become more valuable than anything else, as it gets its hooks into us. 'As addiction develops, the drug increases in metaphorical value,' she says. 'When alcohol occurs to the subcortical brain desperate for relief, financial concerns are utterly dwarfed in significance.'

Makes sense. Back then, two of the most oft-said things about me were 'Cath is smashed again' and 'Cath is shite with money'. And I was. I was a fiscal flibbertigibbet. This manifested itself in several ways.

1. THE UNAUTHORISED OVERDRAFT FEES

I lived in my overdraft from the age of 18 onwards. But it wasn't unnerving *enough* that I lived on the precipice of my overdraft, staring into the howling abyss of no more money. Oh no. Instead, I went headfirst into a ravine of not just minus money, but minus-minus money.

Enter the unauthorised overdraft fee. The most common collection of words on my bank statements. Each month, I would pay at least £100 in these blighters. Why? For those who don't know, this was the ultimate fiscal punishment from your bank. If you went over your overdraft limit, even by a few pounds, you'd encounter the 'bucket of water over the head' of an automatic £25 fine. And there were even sometimes further daily fines thereafter, akin to a financial game of slaps, for every day you remained shivering in the howling abyss.

The reason I would tip over the cliff edge was always, always due to my tandem addictions. Alcohol and its roguish bedfellow tobacco. Whom I would take home for an anxiety-nixing threesome.

Six days from payday, I was always stony broke. But I had a card that would still work for a £12 transaction, despite there being 53p in my account.

So, I would use it. Of course I would.

I would push my card into the off-licence's slot, praying for it to go through. Please, please, please, plastic that feeds my needs. I would spend £12 I didn't have on the second-cheapest bottle of sauvignon blanc (I wasn't a savage) and 10 Marlboro Lights (because I wasn't a smoker, you understand, so I didn't buy 20) and then offset the splurge of those with a 99p pot o' noodles or microwavable pasty. Telling myself that my scrimpin' dinner offset the price of my addictions. *I'm so budget!* Martin Lewis, eat your heart out.

Thwack – a £25 unauthorised overdraft fee. Which meant I'd actually spent £37. For that, I could have had lobster and French fries, Chablis and those gold-tipped candy-coloured cigarettes. *Quelle* dumbass.

From 2006 to 2009, these draconian and daily fines were suspected to be illegal, following some hints dropped by the OFT (Office of Fair Trading). A *Which?* and Money Saving Expert campaign sparked a groundswell – soon a stampede – of Brits then claiming back their cute little bi-yearly fines. 'I claimed back £500 and went on holiday!' case studies would beam out from the local newspaper.

Did I get my act together to claim back my outrageous weekly fines, accrued over six years? Moohaha. You're funny. Did I hell. I was too busy getting shitfaced to fill in a form or two in order to claw back approximately *£8,000*. Eight thousand freakin' pounds! Which, back in 2006, would have been a decent chunk of a deposit for a starter flat in London. Insert crying emoji.

And then in 2009, the money-claimin' fun stopped, when the Supreme Court ruled that such bank charges were actually legal, and OFT had to back off. And with that, my/our window of opportunity for a reclaim snapped shut. Bah. Let's not think about that one too hard, shall we? Moving swiftly on.

2. I WOULD FREELOAD LIKE IT WAS MY JOB
Even colleagues that earned less than me always seemed to be more

flush than me. Thus, surely it was their responsibility to shore me up when I was flailing, no? Gimme. As for those friends who earned more (which was to be fair, most of them), I saw it as their civic duty to keep me in pints of Staropramen in The Nellie Dean.

There were several phases friends cycled through. At first, they would step in like gentlewomen throwing coats over puddles when my card was refused at the bar.

Swoops in 'Please, allow me!' they would say graciously.

Then came the phase of them pointedly sitting there with empty glasses until I offered to buy a round. On occasion, I cried when a friend refused to cover my drink. It seemed a reasonable response. I had no money, she had money, so what in holy heaven was she playing at denying me some pear cider? What monstrous injustice was this?

Some ingenious friends started inserting 'Cashpoint' into our pub crawl, as if it were a destination. Our night would go: The Red Lion, Cashpoint, Bar Soho, Trisha's. 'Let's all get some money out, shall we!' they would rejoice, pointedly withdrawing cash even though they already had tenners stuffed in their wallets, whereas mine was always full of nothing but dust bunnies, a Boot's Advantage card and random buttons.

'Cath, do you need to get some money out?'

The 'Cashpoint' stop was the equivalent of a parent making a big show of washing and drying their hands, in order to be a hand-washing role model for a child. I would stand there stubbornly, kicking my scuffed Dolcis shoes that desperately needed re-heeling against the wall, refusing to get this stupid cash out that they thought was so important.

Oftentimes, I knew full well that I couldn't even withdraw £20. So if the cashpoint was out of £10 notes, I'd face a cringey 'cashpoint say no' moment. *Let's just get to the next bar*, I'd think, clip-clopping around Soho on my worn-out shoes like a steed on clapped-out metal horseshoes.

There, I'd just find men who were willing to buy me drinks. 'Do we have to talk to guys who are thick as breeze-blocks just to get drinks?' my friends would remonstrate. 'We have our own money!'

Speak for yourselves, I would think, while smiling at my next walking cashpoint.

3. I BORROWED MONEY FROM EVERYONE
Seriously, *everyone*.

Just as I would do circuits of off-licences, never hitting the same one too often, I staggered who I asked. The rota generally went: parents, boyfriend, friends and then *even* colleagues.

I once asked the features editor of a magazine I was freelancing on, so *basically my boss for a week*, if I could borrow £20 for a taxi I had idling outside; with a driver that had steam coming out of his ears as well as his exhaust.

You have financial mastery you know not of

When we get sober, we suddenly have a lot more money. Much of that is just simple maths.

Take last night. I had an absolute belter of a night playing Monopoly (The deceit! The cheats! The drama! The hotel-studded gauntlet!) with a few friends. The entire night cost me a grand total of £12 for a tea, a decaf coffee, some fries, and a cake. Ten years ago, this four-hour night out would have segued into an eight-hour night out, and it would've cost me at least £35 including club entry, drunk cheesy chips and a taxi.

As with anything in sobriety, as the years roll by, we can forget to appreciate the shift. The natural savings we're making. We can also accidentally begin spending all that spare money on treats rather than stashing it away.

But here's the thing about being an ex-caner (or a current one who's on the threshold of change). There's financial mastery we know not of, hidden back in the recesses of our brains. You're probably really good at surviving on very little money. Really. We're natural-born cheapskates.

My accountant recently described me as 'very frugal'. I strongly considered printing and framing this email. I take a flask of tea everyplace because I fundamentally object to paying £2.50 for a 10p teabag and hot water. Given I didn't have any 'spare' money for so very long, since I was literally pissing it down the porcelain telephone, I now feel like a sultan for having one takeaway a week. Like Imelda Marcos for spending £50 on a pair of boots. Like Kanye for buying a £500 Ikea bed.

You may relate. 'Luxuries' like takeaways, non-essential footwear and a new mattress that doesn't have stains on it, did not feature in my drinking reality. I couldn't afford those things. Alcohol was sucking up all of my money like an anteater on ants. And so, buying luxuries like a scented candle still feels frivolous.

The upshot is this. Wreckheads do indeed make astonishingly bad financial decisions and waste a fuckload of money. But what's done is done. Meditating on that is a fast lane to madness.

On the flipside, active addiction also means we pick up numerous tricks, side angles and hustles. We're used to living without, after all. We know about discount codes, the bus rather than the train, sales shopping and re-gifting, and how £7 can make a whole week's lunches of pesto pasta.

It's just that, before, we cut these corners to feed a bottomless booze habit, and said habit often had us lobbing all of this budgeting know-how out of the window in order to buy a tray of

Jägerbombs. Now we have our wits about us, we can absolutely make a twenty stretch in the week before payday.

Once we take those skills and run with them, we're better with money than we think. Once we start telling ourselves a different story, the ending changes. Just like taking a DeLorean back to tweak the past, in order to change the future. Dare to change the story you tell yourself. See what happens.

Once I rejected the narrative that I am bad at money, I started getting really good with money. I realised that my fiscal fuckwittery was not an inextricable part of my character; it was a mere offshoot of my addiction. Now, I pay bills early, I file my tax return early, I try to pay for *more* on a night out, if anything.

And now I've bought a flat for the very first time. It wasn't easy, to save a deposit all by my-blinking-self. But I did it. By applying the 'very frugal' luxury-swerving or eking-out philosophies that I learned when I was drinking. And if I can repurpose those skills to save, then you can too. Us boozehounds are better with money than we think we are.

When I was applying for a mortgage, I half expected a big, red, flashing alarm to go off in the financial universe. 'Hell no!' Instead, my application sailed through without a hitch.

And then I realised.

I was applying for a mortgage on the month of my seventh soberversary. And guess how long credit history is stored for, in the UK? Seven years. It felt like fiscal serendipity at its finest.

BURNING QUESTION: CAN YOU HAVE AN 'ADDICTIVE PERSONALITY'?

Dr David Nutt: 'No. And this is an important point to make. People become addicted for different reasons, whether they're predisposed to anxiety, which they self-medicate with alcohol, or they have a stressful, miserable life and seek pleasure in alcohol. There's no single personality type.'

Dr Julia Lewis: 'There is no formal diagnosis of an addictive personality. The best metaphor is of a weighing scales. Certain risk factors – genetics, a chronic pain disorder, trauma – will tip those scales towards "more likely to be addicted." I wouldn't call that "a personality"; it's accumulated risk factors.'

Dr Judith Grisel says: 'Yes. It's incredibly complicated and comes from constellations of tens of thousands of genes. But we know this: those prone to addiction are more likely to be high in novelty-seeking, reward-seeking and risk-taking. We're all about chasing the carrot and less likely to care about the stick.

However, those very same traits are also very useful and can be positives.'

Dr Marc Lewis says: 'We've already discussed how anxiety and introversion can predispose towards addiction, but also the opposite; the tendency towards risk-taking and impulsive behaviour. Given these often contradictory traits can predict the same outcome – an addiction – I believe that means the idea of an "addictive personality" falls by the wayside.

Also, these traits can lead to a whole bunch of possible outcomes. If you have impulsive tendencies, you might become a politician, a mountain climber, a businessperson. Becoming addicted is just one of the possibilities.

What turns that dial of possible outcomes towards addiction is going to be "environmental impact"; the power of childhood experiences and so on. Personality traits are only predispositions, not hard causes.'

IN BED WITH BIG ALCOHOL

Globally, there tends to be a trend of governments colluding with Big Alcohol. Why? Simple, my friend. Money. Alcohol tax revenue makes billions for governments and states worldwide.

Take the UK as an example: alcohol sales made the government between £10.5 and £12.1 billion per annum in the past few years. Yet alcohol also *costs* our government billions. A Public Health England study estimated the total cost to be £21 billion per year – minimum.

Huh? So, it's costing more than it's making? In that case, why aren't our politicians and policymakers *more motivated* to reduce alcohol's impact? Because if alcohol sales fall before the costs 'domino-fall' too (it will take decades for some of the long-term health costs to fall), they're left with a humdinger of a deficit.

If they lose, say £5 billion in a year, and they only recoup £2 billion, you can see the problem. Eventually the loss/costs will even out, and the seesaw will rebalance, but that takes forward-thinking rather than myopic 'What about next year?'

Also, and this cannot be ignored, millions of people's livelihoods depend on bar culture and Big Alcohol. Economic concerns like this are valid, rather than remotely evil, because making a living is inextricably tied to health. And so, we have a star-crossed clusterfuck of a conflict of interest. Which means that, ultimately, I don't think our governments want us to quit drinking. They can't afford it.

Meanwhile, Big Alcohol *certainly* doesn't want that lost profit. 'One estimate is that, if everyone drank within recommended limits, the industry would lose £13 billion,' says Professor David Nutt. That's £13 billion <u>per year</u>. 'That's a lot of lost profit.' Obviously, the drinks industry doesn't want to lose that. Nor does the government. 'Its aim is often aided by the government, which wants the tax income.'

In France: Dry January was cancelled

In 2019, *France 24* reported that the French government actually *cancelled* Dry January after 'intense lobbying' by winemakers. The French alcohol industry complained about the 'total abstinence' the campaign encouraged (even though said encouraged abstinence was *only for one month*). If this doesn't demonstrate the power and sway of the alcohol industry over governmental health decisions, I don't know what does.

'There were backroom decisions taken that raise questions, even though the budgets were set and people were already at work on the campaign,' said Nathalie Latour of Fédération Addiction, in the aforementioned *France 24* article.

In America: Big Alcohol funds medical studies

In 2018, the *New York Times* uncovered a scandal that showed just how insidious Big Alcohol's influence is – even on the health narratives Americans receive about alcohol from their very own National Institute of Health (the equivalent of the NHS). The exposé unveiled documents which proved that, in 2013, an actual federal agency (The National Institute on Alcohol Abuse and Alcoholism) had courted Big Alcohol to fund a $100 million medical study into moderate drinking. Yes, really.

'The documents and interviews show that the Institute waged a vigorous campaign to court the alcohol industry, paying for scientists to travel to meetings with executives, where they gave talks strongly suggesting that the study's results would endorse moderate drinking as healthy,' said the *New York Times*.

This resulting study was more 'marketing' than 'public health research', said Dr Michael Siegel, a professor at Boston University

School of Public Health, in the same piece. No wonder Big Alcohol bit the hands off those who offered up such a study! 'This must have seemed like a dream come true for industry,' added Dr Siegel. 'Of course they would pay for it,' he said. 'They're admitting the trial is designed to provide a justification for moderate drinking. That's not objective science.'

Thankfully, a full investigation followed the *New York Times* piece, and the $100 million study was axed. But if a bloodhound journalist hadn't uncovered who exactly was bankrolling this study, billions of Americans could theoretically have been presented with 'evidence' that daily drinking was a good idea. With no clue that Big Alcohol had sponsored the entire 'study'.

In the UK: the Drinkaware scandal

'Go to Drinkaware for the facts', alcohol labels direct us, citing the website. We obediently trot along, assuming it's an independently run health website. Hello facts!

If you ask your average person: 'Who is behind Drinkaware?' most will say the NHS. Or the government. Or the World Health Organization. Or something of that ilk. People never, ever, unless they're already in the know, guess the reality. That Drinkaware, dispenser of 'the facts' is funded by the alcohol industry itself.

'Drinkaware is a charity funded by the alcohol industry,' confirms Professor David Nutt. On Drinkaware's website itself, it says it is 'funded largely by voluntary and unrestricted donations from UK alcohol producers, retailers and supermarkets.' The Drinkaware Trust calls itself 'independent' and says it's governed by a 'Board of Trustees'.

Yes, you read that right. The body dispensing the information that we are directed to is bankrolled by the very people selling us the booze. It's the likes of Diageo keeping the lights on over at Drinkaware.

Peculiar thing. Drinkaware's national campaigns tend to hinge on one simple concept: keeping Britain chasing moderation. Take the 'alcoholidays' campaign, which endorsed drink-free days for the heaviest-drinking Brits; mid-lifers. Or the 'cut back and feel better' campaign. Or the 'have a little less, feel a lot better' campaign. Etcetera for ever. (The only Drinkaware venture that encouraged *not drinking at all* was the 'Home and Dry' campaign, aimed at drivers.)

I'm going to make a strong statement. You'll never, ever find Drinkaware rolling out a national campaign that encourages anything but moderation. If there is ever a 'quit drinking and feel better!' Drinkaware campaign, I'll officially eat my bobble hat with a side of kimchi.

Why? Drinkaware ultimately doesn't want Britain to quit drinking, given who pays the electricity bill. Its modus operandi is 'harm reduction' or having more alcohol-free days. Which seems noble at first glance, until you think about where that message is ultimately coming from. It wants Britain to chase moderation, *ad infinitum*. Because: ker-ching!

When I tell people about this link, this buried bankrolling, this health website masquerading, their reaction is always of this ilk: 'How crooked is that? The nepotism!' That would be like a fizzy-drink producer setting up a shell 'charity' and calling it 'Sugaraware' and directing unsuspecting consumers to its website, rather than to an independent, non-biased health website. 'Go to Sugaraware for the facts!' it would say on the drink cans.

Yet, we live in some parallel universe where the industries that cause untold mental – and physical – damage somehow provide 'the facts' to the public. It feels a little like Biff's dystopian ruled realm in

Back to the Future II, no? The British Medical Association said back in 2012 that, 'The involvement of the Drinkaware Trust in providing public health communications is a significant area of concern.'

An expert-penned paper entitled 'Be Aware of Drinkaware' said, 'Although the British addiction field and the wider public health community have distanced themselves from the Portman Group, they have not done so from Drinkaware, even though Drinkaware was devised by the Portman Group to serve industry interests. Both long-standing and more recent developments indicate very high levels of industry influence on British alcohol policy.'

In April 2019, an insider told me that the health world was 'pretty furious' about a statement the Portman Group released referring to the 'risks' of alcohol consumption. The inverted commas are an affront because they suggest the *risks* are debatable, when they're undeniable. The latest figures from the Office of National Statistics said that British alcohol-specific deaths in 2017 totalled 21 deaths per day. To say 'risks' is an insult.

Alcohol labels pointing toward Drinkaware are an absolute disgrace. In 2018, The Royal Society for Public Health called the alarming public blind spot around the risks of drinking an 'awareness vacuum'. And back in 2017, 25 health leaders signed a public letter saying that labelling on alcohol ought to point towards the NHS website instead – what a fine idea!

Drinkaware is performative. It's not unlike a company fulfilling its corporate social responsibility by sending all of its workers on a mindfulness course. Relax! And then continuing to run a culture of expected 60-hour weeks.

The name of the study we talked about said it best. Be aware of Drinkaware. Or should it be: *Beware of Drinkaware.* The wolf in sheep's clothing, that's somehow been allowed into a field that it has absolutely no place in.

Why is the drinks industry even in the room?

It's bigger than just Drinkaware and the UK. Drinkaware is the mere tip of the global iceberg. The collusion between our governments and the industry is promiscuous in the extreme.

Last year, the *Guardian* ran a headline entitled 'Alcohol industry fingerprints all over Australia's plan to tackle overdrinking'. You guessed it – it's all about how Big Alcohol Oz influences the federal government there. 'It's quite remarkable how politicians and governments want to cosy up to the alcohol industry', Michael Thorn of FARE (Foundation for Alcohol Research and Education) told the *Guardian* Australia. 'Yes, donations are part of explaining that.' As in, political donations from Big Alcohol.

Take one shocking story (of many) that Professor Nutt tells in his book *Drink: the new science of alcohol + your health*. I'll nutshell it for you. In 2010, the Department of Health set up a group (the RDAN) to encourage people to drink within the recommended guidelines. 'The problem was, the government decided this group was to be made up of 50 per cent health experts and 50 per cent representatives of the drinks industry', Professor Nutt says.

Wrap your head around that. A health group created by the British government to reduce the harms of alcohol, that is half composed of the *people who profit from the alcohol*. It was as farcical as it sounds. By 2011, all of the health experts had quit. There was simply no point in the committee existing. 'It was clearly impossible to be objective when half the committee had a specific link to the industry that was causing the problem,' says Professor Nutt.

'The drinks industry wants you to keep drinking. That is its reason for existing,' says Professor Nutt. 'When it comes to deciding how to prevent the harms of alcohol, the drinks industry doesn't even have a right to be in the room.' And yet it so often *is in the room*.

When the WHO advised restricting alcohol access

In April 2020, after the outbreak of the global pandemic, the World Health Organization issued strongly worded advice that governments worldwide should 'enforce measures which limit alcohol consumption'. Not only because it makes people more vulnerable to contracting Covid-19, but also because it increases the incidence of violent behaviour, such as domestic abuse.

Many countries listened up. In places such as Thailand, South Africa and India, alcohol sales were outlawed, in order to keep hospital beds free for Covid-19 patients. It wasn't a perfect strategy. Maybe too extreme. These 1920s Prohibition-style bans inevitably lead to bootlegging and speakeasies. In Mexico, there were around 70 deaths from people drinking moonshine. Why? Outright bans push those who are addicted underground.

But at least these countries were placing national health over alcohol-related GDP. What's more, it worked, in keeping hospitals clear(er). The proof? In South Africa, once they lifted the ban, Emergency Room visits doubled.

Over in Britain, they may as well have doused the WHO advice in vodka and burned it. First off, they made off-licences 'essential'. Huh? Over in the USA it made sense to keep liquor stores open during the lockdowns, since in many states, that's pretty much the only place you can buy it. Addicted drinkers can go into savage withdrawal without booze.

But in the UK, making off-licences* 'essential' was a farce. Given

---

* International readers, you may not know what an off-licence is, so allow me: off-licences are purely dedicated bottle shops, often in or on the outskirts of cities, often expansive, and they're the place you go for a rare wine, a specialist vodka or a craft ale. If you live someplace remote, you're almost definitely closer to a village shop or a supermarket (that will sell lots of alcohol) than an off-licence.

every other 'essential' shop in the UK stocks alcohol plentifully too – namely supermarkets, corner shops and petrol stations. As a result of the government's protection of alcohol off-licence sales – or indeed panic stockpiling – Nielsen reported that March alone saw a 67 per cent surge in alcohol profits.

Come July 2020, the British government re-opened pubs before health-promoting, immune-system-boosting services such as gyms, yoga studios and leisure centres. As well as alternative socialising hubs such as soft-play centres or bowling alleys. Even libraries and schools (for all ages) were re-opened later than pubs. In doing so, the government makes its priorities clear. Boozing over fitness! Alcohol over learning!

'The British government's actions have raised concerns about the level of influence the alcohol industry has on policy. Mr Wetherspoon seems to be quite an influencer,' says Dr Julia Lewis. Meanwhile, Americans were given different messages altogether, with the CDC advising them to avoid alcohol during celebrations such as Thanksgiving. What a curious transatlantic contradiction.

Teetotalling is a political tinderbox

Now we know about the economic engine that drives political decisions about alcohol policy. But in Britain at least, we also have this: MPs are reportedly uncommonly fond of the lash themselves. At Westminster, there are 16 bars and restaurants on-site, and receptions where free alcohol flows, making it probably the most alcohol-available workplace in the land.

British MPs officially drink more than your average person, said a 2020 study published in the *British Medical Journal*. The research found a 'higher proportion of MPs with risky drinking' than your regular citizen. Dr Dan Poulter, a psychiatrist and MP, told the *Guardian*: 'It is extraordinary that there are so many bars in parliament where alcohol is available at almost every hour of the day. This is not the case in other parliaments elsewhere in the world.' Or other workplaces, he hastens to add.

This boozy workplace will undoubtedly be influencing the decisions MPs make about our access to alcohol as a nation. Because, after all, if have a penchant for doing something yourself, aren't you more likely to vote to keep that thing going?

***

As you can see, the sober revolution is an economic – and therefore a political – tinderbox, since it threatens to torch billions of tax revenue. Many sober uprisings are squelched, given the tug o' war between health and money. Of course, I don't wish poverty on our governments or states – many of those tax coffers are used for good rather than nonsense politician expenses. But one thing's for sure. When deciding upon issues of health + alcohol, Big Alcohol needs to stop being allowed into the room, let alone into the bed.

It's funny, isn't it, how drinking is still seen as radical, rebellious – like wearing a leather jacket and an arched eyebrow astride a motorbike – even though it's the pedestrian norm. Given all that we've just discussed, opting out on drinking is actually a one-finger-salute to The Man.

It's sticking it to the moguls who sit in leather boardroom recliners and still dictate so much of the messaging we receive. *Who still want us to drink*, no matter what they say in limp-wristed health warnings. This makes teetotalling one of the most punk things you can do.

30 THINGS I'VE LEARNED
ABOUT BOUNDARIES

It's a truth universally acknowledged that, in order to get and stay sober, you need something called 'boundaries'.

Know what these are? You probably do, you clever badger, but I'm going to spell it out anyway, because before recovery, I thought these were exclusively the stuff of property delineation disputes.

Boundaries are invisible lines, usually drawn out by a 'no, I can't do that', where you denote what you are and are not willing to do. They sketch out a border around you so that you can protect your time, physical space, wellbeing, emotions, money; all that good stuff. 'This is my dance space, this is your dance space', essentially.

Boundaries are essential to feeling safe in long-term recovery. Why? They keep your sanity ring-fenced from others. Here's what I've learned. In the order of learning it.

1. I hate boundaries!
2. I need boundaries.
3. I hate boundaries! Life would be so much easier if I just did what other people wanted of me.
4. I need boundaries.
   Otherwise I will be cannibalised from the inside by resentment. Resentment that my time and energy is not my own.
5. The first time you say, 'No, I can't do that', you will feel like sliding down a wall, scrunching yourself into a tiny ball, rocking, and going 'eeeeeeee'. (Or you may *literally* do that, like I did.) The discomfort will be astronomical. Oosh.

6. Those who are *not* people-pleasers do not struggle to set boundaries. They don't even know what 'boundaries' are. They just call that 'responding'.

7. Ergo, if you struggle with this too, you are probably a people-pleaser. I know! I didn't think I was a people-pleaser either, until – boundaries.

8. There will be an 'I am a bad person' hangover after you start setting boundaries. It will linger. (Especially when you lay them down with family. Something primordial within us always wants to say 'yes' to family.)

9. You will rewrite text messages numerous times because you feel like an egomaniac. You will feel selfish, arrogant and awkward, even when being spectacularly reasonable.

10. Shoe-switching helps. If somebody said this exact same thing to you, would you consider them to be an imperious narcissist? Well then.

11. You will feel a knee-jerk urge to apologise profusely, for saying you cannot do this favour, or talk right now, or meet this tight deadline, or pick up that thing, or attend this event, or [insert thing asked of you].

12. *You have not done anything wrong.* You have not done anything wrong. Really, you need to tattoo this on the insides of your eyelids during the advent of boundary-setting.

13. Saying 'no' is not a criminal offence, a transgression, or a social taboo. Don't apologise, if you can bear it.* Why? Apologising perpetuates the notion in the other person's (and your) eyes that when you say 'no', you have done something wrong.

---

* British readers, I realise this is a Big Ask given we apologise approximately 29 times a day for simply existing.

14. 'I'm afraid I'll have to say no' is a good, softly couched happy medium.

15. Womxn tend to have a harder time setting boundaries given they are generally raised, socially conditioned, or culturally expected to be helpful, compliant and endlessly generous of their time and energy.

16. In a perfect world, where I would have a pony in my garden, plus a glass elevator and a spa in my residence (is that Binary Barbie's dream house?), nobody ought to press on our 'no's to make them crack.

17. This is not a perfect world. People won't just press – they will jump up and down on your 'no's like they're a bloody trampoline.

18. Some of your most woke friends, who will nod solemnly in agreement with your boundary-setting, will hear a silent addendum.
    'I can't socialise mid-week any more *except for with you.*'
    'I can't do any playdates in the near future, *except for with your children.*'
    'I'm not lending anyone money any more, *except for you.*'
    'I like to run alone, *except for with you.*'

19. They will then take the silent 'exception' addendum that only they heard and crowbar themselves into your next run, or try to schedule a playdate, or ask to borrow a tenner, or, or, or.

20. You will then need to re-boundary, because they were hearing things that were not there. You may need to write your boundary in a neon ten-foot sign and plonk them in front of it.

21. 'Blind to boundary-setting' people are most likely those who have very permeable boundaries themselves. It's like

Hanlon's Razor, but blunted: 'Never attribute to malice that which can be explained by ~~stupidity~~ obliviousness.'

22. The oblivious (of which I was once one; weren't you?) were probably also never taught that it's OK to say 'no'. Summon compassion. While also: Spelling. It. Out. 'Kind, light and polite' is my go-to style guide.

23. But then, there are also people who hear your 'no', but disrespect it anyhow. One of the most common ways a boundary disrespecter will drive a monster truck over your boundary is by pretending you never said anything, or that they misheard. 'You said not to come by?' they'll say, having shown up at your house. 'I thought you said not to bring pie!'

24. Does your boundary make this person angry? Do they hurl 'selfish' at you because you dared to say no? It's a cliché because it's true. Those who benefited the most from your lack of boundaries will be those most affronted by the erection of them. They're angry because they were previously breakdancing all over your lack of boundaries, and now you've thrown up a fence that has ruined their fun.

25. There's also the ultra passive-aggressive 'So you have time to' crew.
    'So you have time to post on social media, but not call me?'
    'So you have time to work out, but not help me?'
    This is a red flag because it's a dead giveaway that 'So you have time to' feels a misguided proprietorship over *your* time. Which would be like a neighbour scaling your wall to sunbathe in your garden.

26. Pre-boundaries, your time/energy scoreboard looked like this:
    Everyone else: 2
    You: 0

27. Post-boundarics, it will ideally look like this:
    You: 1
    Everyone else: 1
28. This isn't a case of never *doing anything for anyone else ever*, or saying no to everything, or telling your friends and family to go hang. That's a fast route to becoming an island of a person. It's a case of making sure you have half left for yourself, once you're done bestowing that which you can happily, generously spare.
29. Let's all please agree to teach our kids, nieces, nephews, younger cousins and the kid who lives next door that boundaries are healthy, not selfish. A better world beckons, if we can do this!*
30. Feel free to say 'no' to #29's mission if you don't have time/energy. I respect you all the more for it. You boundary-setting baller.

'Walls keep everybody out.
Boundaries teach people where the door is.'

Mark Groves

---

* I want to talk about a 'new dawn', but that's verging on a vampire romance.

THE LGBTQIA COMMUNITY ON SOBERING UP

This chapter came about by accident. I sent out a bat-signal on Instagram, calling for men to tell me about their experiences of being sober (you can read this on pages 167–8) Given I didn't want it to be 2D hetero and binary Tarzan-swingin' nonsense, I actively encouraged those from the LGBTQIA community to contribute.

What I didn't expect was to be deluged by the LGBTQIA community at large on how much harder it is to recover within it. Say what? *I did not know that.*

Yep. It turns out that a movement whose defining Big Bang inception occurred in a bar (I discover The Stonewall Inn is literally called 'mecca') is naturally very bloody boozy. Even in today's supposedly progressive society, I'm told that LGBTQ+ bars and nightclubs are the only 'safe' places to flirt and, thus, alcohol becomes an inextricable part of coming out and dating.

I'm told that given these bars and clubs were the portals to freedom of expression from the outset, they are not only symbolic of belonging, they're literal hubs. The centres of the LGBTQ+ community in any town. Which means that when you no longer frequent them as much (or at all), you start to feel frozen out. You feel like you've not just 'lost' alcohol or your drug of choice, you've also 'lost' that community.

Woah. I had no idea. This saddens me. Here are some stories I was told:

'On one hand, going to gay bars and clubs as a young person can be a rite of passage that is wonderful and life-affirming. It allows people to feel accepted – possibly for the first time in life. On the other hand, unfortunately, it also normalises excessive drinking.'

Cole

'The whole LGBTQ+ community started in bars and clubs. Gay pride in NYC centres upon the bars around The Stonewall Inn; a bar where the gay movement started. I was a bartender in one said bar for many years in my twenties, serving in underwear only. The first thing you receive at a dinner party is some exotic, expensive, high-alcohol drink. Now that I've turned 50, most of the people I know collect wine or whiskey. The more expensive the better. Alcohol is like church in the gay community: full of ceremony and bringing redemption because you forget fears and anger. I would tell friends, "I'm worried that I'm drinking every day", and they would say – "us too. No big deal." I feel so much better now I'm sober. Honestly, it boiled down to vanity for me. It was affecting my looks!'

Harry

'When I was younger and battling with being gay, I relied heavily on alcohol to numb my inhibitions around other guys. I couldn't dance, flirt with or kiss another man without being incredibly drunk. When you're new to the LGBTQ+ scene, it feels awkward, embarrassing and very exposing to do it fully present and sober. It's hard to get sober and still feel connected to the community – *but it is possible*.'

Sam

'Most gay social events are in bars. I mean, you can go to those and not drink. But at 11pm I'd rather be in bed than on a poorly lit dance floor listening to Lady Gaga remixes and drinking flat Coke.'

Nia

'I presented as a gay dude forever, but was always very uncomfortable in my own skin. I never had a first date that led to sexy times without being at least gently drunk, but generally shitfaced. I might have had a *fifteenth* date sober, but I was probably still hungover. I was scared of all sorts of things, but the more drunk I was, the more I could ignore it. Just after getting sober, two people directly asked me if I was trans. Fuck. Couldn't ignore the question or answer any more. The answer was yes. I'm non-binary trans femme and have now been out for 11 months, and sober for 13 months. It's not always easy, but it is always worth it.'

Alex

'I quit drinking at 33 and am only just beginning to understand how alcohol was a coping mechanism for both a) coming to terms with my sexuality and b) homophobia and heteronormative expectations. Alcohol is central to going out and finding your 'people', so when you stop drinking, it can feel like cutting yourself off. Maybe we need a queer sober movement?'

Anna

- Looking for teetotal LGBTQIA community? Club Soda runs events through 'Queers without Beers' (follow @QWB_UK) and in the US 'Gay and Sober' organises meet-ups (@gayandsober).

PARTIES ARE EXPENSIVE

Let's not pretend alcohol has no flipside. It does. For real. It takes jewel-coloured veils and dances them between you and your most anxious self. It is a legal, easy way to medicate that low thrum of nervousness that most of us (all of us?) feel before a big party.

It works, yes. In the short-term. But there's a steep price to pay. It's a Faustian pact. And that price just gets steeper the longer and deeper in you go. Over years of use, it starts to exacerbate, rather than soothe, your anxiety.

For a socially anxious introvert, as many recoverees are, early teen years are oftspent feeling adrift from inclusion and togetherness in large groups. We find that click of connection one-on-one, but faced with a roomful? It's like we're bobbing on a boat at sea, watching Lego-sized people dance at a party on the shore. For a while, alcohol works as a tug rope to bring the little boat in.

But the more we use that tug rope; the harder we pull on it, the more it frays. The tug rope stops working, which means that when drunk, we can feel utterly, profoundly, existentially alone, even with friends. In blackout bedlam? Our boat and us sink into the inky unfathomables.

When we quit drinking, we flee that Faustian pact. But it's no understatement to say that getting sober means we have to learn to socialise all over again. We're newborn hatchlings. A wet kitten. A knobbly-kneed calf. It's abominably exhausting and discombobulating. While also being enormously worthwhile.

I don't know one – one! – ex-drinker who would tell you they find parties easy. Why? Because parties aren't easy. The reason they feel easier when we're loaded is because we've poured a social-anxiety numbing agent into ourselves.

Sober, we learn that parties are expensive. That they cost a king's ransom of energy. That even a coffee with a new friend demands a princely sum. That a date is to ransack a princess's jewels. In early sobriety, we learn to spend discriminately, carefully, rarely, until it's no longer as expensive.

Here are some of the beautiful perks – and differences – of partying sunshine warm sober.

STONE COLD DRUNK	SUNSHINE WARM SOBER
I slather myself in come-get-me-boyz scent.	I put on my relaxing aromatherapy roll-on. My readiment for stepping out into the sooty shawl of night is about me, not them.
I'll pee anywhere. In any slummy dunny. I'll even wee outside, behind trees or rows of shops, when I'm truly batfaced.	In manky pub loos, I build origami loo-seat covers out of single sheets and master the art of ablutions without using my hands.
Free-flowing, cheap booze is the priority. Artisan cocktails are the enemy, given they suck up all of my drinking money.	Food and music become enormously relevant. Board games feel sent from heaven. Open fires or pretty gardens are a major draw.

STONE COLD DRUNK	SUNSHINE WARM SOBER
I hold lavish three-course dinner parties, where I pretend to be a fully functioning grown-up by stuffing a mushroom. I preen about in a Cath Kidston apron and present my latest inedible, lopsided baking.	You'll get one course (and *maybe* some shop-bought ice cream; baking's not my strength) and it might even be served on a tray, if we're feeling casual. The food will be better, the chat less contrived, and I won't be inexplicably wearing high heels in my actual home. You won't leave mine legless because I've insisted on topping up your glass, even when you begged me not to.
Drinking Me at a friend's 30th once: 'A friend and I are going to blow this party off, it's lame,' I said to a mutual friend in the toilets. Cattiness: maximum. I then wondered why the birthday girl (who was no doubt told of this mutiny, where I tried to lead people away from her birthday like some nefarious pied piper) was mysteriously busy forevermore.	Even if your party is the lamest party in the history of parties; if it's your birthday, or your housewarming, or your anything, and I love you, I will find things to like about it, no matter what.

STONE COLD DRUNK	SUNSHINE WARM SOBER
Next day: If it was a weekend, I'd usually tactically keep it clear, in case moving made me vomit in my own mouth a little bit. (Is it just me, or is the sky caving in?) If I erroneously make plans, I either cancel them or wince and fake-smile my way through them.	Next day: It's just a regular day in which I can do everything I normally would. I've not hobbled myself with booze. Get cape, wear cape, fly.

'I've heard a lot of smart people say again and again that they "lost their drinking privilege". Let's get clear on this: It is not a privilege to "be able to" ingest a substance that's sabotaging your health and spirit and life in a hundred different ways.'

Holly Whitaker,
Quit Like a Woman

THE PROBLEMATIC
LANGUAGE AROUND
THE PROBLEM

'You suppose you are the trouble, but you are the cure.
You suppose that you are the lock on the door.
But you are the key that opens it.'

Rumi

There's an insidious trend in the lexicon we use around alcohol addiction. A trend for making us the bad guys and alcohol the innocent party. A trend for sending us up to the dock, and depicting alcohol as the plaintiff. *Poor alcohol.*

The 'problem' of alcohol being our most common addiction is not solely down to the person holding the alcohol. The 'problem drinker'. We're not absolved of responsibility, heck no, given it most certainly takes two to tango. But what the language around addiction glosses over, dances around and distracts us from is: there's <u>a problem </u>with all of it.

The problem of alcohol addiction is not only personal, it's also systemic, cultural, political, capitalistic and social. In most societies, we're expected to grow up to be drinkers, then we're peer-pressured and marketed into drinking regularly. We're repeatedly told non-drinking is a non-life; we're urged to chase moderation and somewhere along the way we get hooked *because it's addictive.*

Then we fear quitting because we fear much of the language we're going to talk about right now. We fear the subtle, or not-so-subtle, implication that when we develop an alcohol dependence, it's all our fault, our failing and nothing to do with the aforementioned constellation of factors that stimulated our addiction into being.

In two words. Fuck that.

Drink responsibly

'Drink responsibly', the labels slapped on British bottles of booze, have rightfully become a national joke. Memes go viral saying things like, 'To me, drink responsibly means: don't spill it'. Or the meme of *Mad Men*'s Don Draper cradling a whiskey sour and saying 'Drink responsibly? Shiiit. Responsibility is *why* I drink.'

(Meanwhile, real Jon Hamm checked into rehab for alcohol addiction before *Mad Men* wrapped.)

The very nature of booze means you become irresponsible. So 'drink responsibly' is a paradox. And why is the alcohol absolved of all responsibility? We don't have signs on wet floors saying 'Walk responsibly' or labels on cigarettes saying 'Smoke responsibly'. Why? Wet floors and cigarettes acknowledge that if peril befalls you, then they are partially to blame. Not wholly, but partially. Given they have mopped the floor you are walking on, or marketed, manufactured and sold the product to you.

'Drink responsibly' is a very clever sleight of hand that enables Big Alcohol to shunt the blame onto the drinker. 'Oh no! You misused our luxury product! We told you to be responsible! Bad bunny!' It's their way of wriggling out from under the responsibility of widespread alcohol harm. It's maddening.

Alcohol abuse

'Alcohol abuse' and 'drug abuse' are the two worst offenders, language-wise. The arrangement of the phrase conjures to mind 'animal abuse' and 'child abuse'. Ergo, 'alcohol abuse' makes it sound as if we are dragging whimpering ale in a choke-collar to a dogfight, or grooming vodka by offering it an ice cream and luring it into a vehicle.

We're apparently 'alcohol abusers' when we drink too much of it. Yet, alcohol is an addictive drug and, thus, it's inevitably moreish. Saying that drinking lots of alcohol is *abusing* it makes it sound like we are terrible people and alcohol is our victim. Which, given Big Alcohol is a billion-pound industry that wants us to drink their product, would be like saying that spending thousands in a clothes shop is abusing it. 'Clothes-shop abuse!' Oh, poor Mango! We need to protect Mango, you diabolical abuser, you.

Yes, your overuse of the clothes shop is self-sabotage, but the clothes shop is not being *abused* by you. You're not calling the clothes shop a tosspot and giving it a kick up the ass. That's abuse. Spending lots of money there is not.

We don't say 'cigarette abuse' or 'casino abuse' because we acknowledge that with smoking and gambling, there is a capitalist megastructure benefiting from our use of those addictive substances and pursuits. The alcohol industry has played a blinder in making us forget that they're culpable. The main thing we're abusing when we drink lots of alcohol is ourselves. Thus, it should be called 'Yourself abuse', all things considered.

Mercifully, the connotations of 'alcohol abuse' have not gone unnoticed. A few years ago, it was watered down to become 'misuse of alcohol'. Now, the term *du jour* is 'alcohol use disorder'. Why the change?

A groundbreaking 2010 study proved that saying 'abuser' rather than 'use disorder' dimmed the view of even those who are sworn to remain objective; 500 mental-health clinicians. Describing a client as an 'abuser' (rather than a person with a 'use disorder') made the clinicians more inclined to think that addiction was due to a flawed character. And to recommend that 'punitive measures' ought to be taken against them.

So, it's not an irrational leap to suggest that in a court of law, should someone be described as a 'substance abuser' rather than 'a person with a substance use disorder' they might actually get time in jail, rather than community service.

Language matters, hugely. Thank you, addiction experts, for kicking 'alcohol abuse' out and introducing 'alcohol use disorder'. It helps.

Normies

In The Rooms (as we colloquially call AA meetings), it's very common to refer to those who can moderate as 'normies'. It's used in various ways; often with a smear of sadness. Oh, those lucky normies, who haven't blown up their drinking privileges! Or with a crack of wry wit.

I'm as partial to a normie joke as anyone – 'my boyfriend started this bottle of wine on Wednesday; it's now Sunday and he still hasn't finished it. This normie doesn't know how to drink *at all*!'

But I now find myself questioning this received language, given the eradication of discrimination hinges upon:

1. Recognising we are all, at our core, the same. We're just humans.

2. The binning of polarising and negative language.

'Normie' is clearly polarising and negative, given there's a clear sidestep that a non-normie is indeed an 'abnormie' (I know, I know, I'm so smart that I figured that one out all by myself. *Twirls hair*).

So given the 'abnormal' subtext, I wonder why we use it at all? What the heck are we doing?! We're colluding in language that does us a disservice. Even if it does make for some fun jokes. 'Look at that normie, leaving half of their wine; *quelle horreur*!'

There are, of course, people who are not remotely preoccupied with alcohol, whose minds award it the same significance as lemonade. You'll know these people because they sometimes genuinely forget you don't drink.

One of these rare-as-snow-leopards people once tried to give me a bottle of wine for Christmas when I was five years sober. He knew I didn't drink, he'd even been on holiday with me twice, but he just... forgot. I stood there holding the bottle of shiraz and said, 'Thank you, T, but what am I gonna do with this – use it as a doorstop?'

'Oh my, I totally forgot!' he cried, swiping the bottle back off me as if I was in mortal danger. But it was funny. He's not a 'normie' and I'm not an 'abnormie'. We're just both humans, one of whom has been addicted to alcohol; one of whom has not. End of.

There's also the interesting curveball that you most definitely don't need to be addicted to alcohol to die from the consumption of it. 'Normies' die too. Even if you're a five or a six on that one-to-ten spectrum of addiction, rather than a seven or up.

Liver specialist Dr Nick Sheron has revealed that, 'only around one third of our patients with alcohol-related cirrhosis have severe alcohol dependency.' The remaining two-thirds? Are 'heavy social drinkers'. Really wrap your head around that: two-thirds of those who end up on a liver ward are *not classified as addicted.*

What's the difference between a 'heavy social drinker' and an 'addicted drinker'? How do you qualify who is a 'normie' and who is not? This is a problem. Largely, it's left to self-identification.

Given this, I wonder if the black-and-white thinking around

'alcoholic' and 'normie' is actually meaning people such as these drink their way into an early grave. I'm sure the 'I'm not an alcoholic, though!' get-out kept this two-thirds of patients drinking, and thus sliding towards chronic illness. We need to see that there are innumerable shades of grey, and binary language isn't helping that.

Alcoholic / Addict

And now, we come to the most hotly debated terms of all. Brace yourselves, buddies. We're going in.

This is a watershed moment in the sobersphere. Can you feel it? Largely, treatment modalities and the lexicon of addiction have remained unchanged since the 1930s, when AA was born and proffered an empathetic refuge for the stigmatised. But in the past decade, the tectonic plates of treatment and language have shifted. A clear desire to move away from labels is present.

There is no specific research into whether labels like 'alcoholic' and 'addict' aid recovery. The only way we can get an overview of it is by looking at programmes that encourage labels (such as AA – more on this in a moment) and those that don't use labels at all.

So let's take a look at some non-labelling alternative programmes, such as Women for Sobriety, LifeRing and SMART. News just in says their efficacy is comparable. A 2018 study discovered that, 'WFS, LifeRing, and SMART are as effective as 12-step groups for those with AUDs [alcohol use disorders].'

Newcomers such as Tempest (personalised online recovery) and Refuge Recovery (a Buddhism-based programme) have now joined our midst and, similarly, they don't endorse labels. But the confrontation of addiction is the same – in Refuge Recovery, the programme 'begins with accepting the reality of our addiction'.

Denial – pierced. Acceptance – gained. Recovery – started. (I haven't seen any data comparing the efficacy of these two newbies with AA yet.)

The irony is, AA purists would tell you that nobody ought to feel pressure to use a label in an AA meeting either. If chaired properly, newcomers should be reminded of this wriggle room. Co-founder Bill W himself said in a 1946 essay for *The Grapevine* that, 'He* doesn't even have to admit that he is an alcoholic.'

This roomy-mindedness has mostly been lost in the mists of time. That wasn't my lived experience in meetings. When 25 other people have introduced themselves as alcoholics, and you dig for the courage to stick your hand up, and all eyes swivel to you, and your mouth opens – it just falls out. The irresistible pull of the 'herding' effect kicks in. I didn't introduce myself as an 'alcoholic' during the first few meetings; afterwards, kind fellows talked to me about denial and acceptance.

The only time I heard anyone stray from this script in 75+ meetings was... let's call him Callum. Who said, 'My name's Callum, today I'm 36 years sober and I'm a recovered alcoholic.' As a newborn, I thought, *"Oh Callum, don't you know you're never recovered! You're going down, my friend!"* I thought Callum was swaddled in layers of pride, ego and denial. I had about six days sober at the time, so what the hell did I know? Nowadays, I would high-five him for knowing his own mind and choosing his own lexicon. We're allowed to.

I still say I'm in recovery, and probably will for ever, but I don't know how I'll feel after 36 years, so who am I to presume to tell Callum what to do/think?!

---

* Bill forgot to mention she/they as well as 'he', the silly sausage.

The label comes with relief

Back in 2013, I did feel *that* overwhelming sense of relief the first time I said, 'My name's Catherine and I'm an alcoholic,' in a meeting. That's undeniable. I'd named my issue and set the machinery in motion for my recovery. Finally, I could stop pretending to be OK. Finally, the healing could begin.

But now I wonder if those exact words were necessary, or if, 'My name's Catherine and I'm addicted to alcohol,' would have been just as profound and powerful. A person addicted to a thing, rather than a person *as* an addiction.

The reason I ponder and wonder this more and more is because I see:

a) Evidence that the stigma surrounding 'addict' and 'alcoholic' is alive and kicking, even in today's woke society. There are several sources listed in the back that confirm this, if you're interested.

b) Evidence that shows that the aforementioned stigma around the 'for ever' labelling puts people off seeking help. They don't want the stigma so, frankly, they carry on drinking and using. Not good.

c) The groundswell of younger generations successfully getting sober and streaking into long-term recovery, without the use of any labels whatsoever (around half of my readers report having gotten sober without using a label).

d) Zero evidence that less emotive labels such as 'teetotal' and 'non-drinker' carry the same negative stigma.

Fearmongering folklore surrounds the rejection of labels, but I've never seen any hard proof that they are necessary. Have you? Label rejectionists are marked with a 'Relapse Pending' label and dismissed. But nobody sticks around to see if they might actually *not* relapse.

A game-changer for me was reading that the backbone of Tempest's personalised recovery programme is thus: 'Addiction is an experience, not an identity.' WOAH. Hearing that made me feel like I'd had my brain removed, zhushed and placed back in my head, at a slightly different angle.

The lexicon trapdoor

I started eyeballing the word 'alcoholic' back in 2017 and nudging it towards the edge of my lexicon trapdoor. I didn't tell anyone about this; my squinting at the word. I still said 'Yup!' if someone asked me if I was an alcoholic. Nonetheless, I stopped thinking about myself as an alcoholic, just to see.

Why did I do it in secret? Because, as mentioned, I'd been taught that taking off the word was like shrugging on the showy garments of ego, pride and denial instead. *Does a twirl and moves closer to a drink.*

I was taught that offloading 'alcoholic' was akin to flipping a switch to start the grind and growl of the relapse machine. So even *considering* offloading it made me slightly nervous. I half expected to burst into flames of need, upon which I would be forced to run to the nearest establishment (a bar, natch) for them to douse me with the nearest bucket of something (cider slops, of course).

Or maybe a dancing red dot would appear on my forehead while I obliviously folded washing; meanwhile a sobriety-slaying sniper would hunker down into position to take their shot. I would be marked for neutralising.

Guess what: after some initial nervousness around it, nothing happened. What a giant anti-climax. If anything, I felt safer in my sobriety. I'm not saying that will be the same experience for everyone, and I was four years sober at the time. But I'm telling you this because it's true and it was *not* what I expected.

Rearranging deck chairs on the Titanic

Where did I get these ideas, that removing 'alcoholic' would put me in such danger? Many, many cautionary tales in meetings, but also the following conversation with my father:

Me: 'I've just read this book by this Jason Vale guy who says that you can quit drinking, and stay sober, without calling yourself an alcoholic.'

Him: 'Well, we'll see how Jason feels about that when he starts drinking again.'

It was a short, sharp slap-down. No questioning of the pre-approved vocabulary! You'll wind up face down in a pitcher of beer, dear. It's no great mystery, is it, that I got the message that 'alcoholic' was a necessary part of the narrative arc. That semantics-resisting would be as insane as rearranging deckchairs on the Titanic. And so I toed the line and said what I was told to.

A curious quirk. Whenever you tentatively suggest that labels maybe aren't necessary, that maybe you no longer identify as an alcoholic, the giant leap of assumption is often thus: *you are considering drinking again*. Even though you said no such thing!

And yet: 'I no longer identify as an alcoholic because I'm not currently addicted to alcohol' and 'I'm now going to go out and get twatted on red wine!' are two galactically different things.

I know I'm not currently addicted to alcohol because I could literally live six feet away from wine (and have done so) and not want to drink it. But that doesn't mean that I don't know that my addictive neural superhighways are still buried in my brain, albeit covered in cobwebs and dust bunnies from many years of disuse.

Abstinence is the antidote to active addiction; creating new 'non-drinking' neural pathways. But it can never remove those deep-down neural pathways of previous addiction. Which is why I no more nurse the chimera of moderation than I would nurse the notion that I can outrun lions.

You don't need to wear an identifying label forevermore to remind you of this neuroscientific fact. 'I'm not currently addicted' + 'I know I would most likely be addicted again if I picked up', are two things that *can and do* co-exist. To suggest they can't is an insult to our intelligence. As if we're going to *forget* that we were once addicted to alcohol. As if it'll *slip our minds* that we probably shouldn't play with that particular loaded gun.

People-first language

Coming back to the aforementioned evidence of a) and b), changes are afoot. Knowing that the labels come with a side of stigma, and can act as a barrier for seeking help, addiction experts and bodies are increasingly pushing for 'people-first' language.

Most notably The National Institute of Health, but numerous others besides. 'X has an alcohol dependence' or 'Y was addicted to' is now the language of choice. Even some scientific addiction journals now refuse to use 'addiction-as-identity' language.

Meanwhile, a parallel reality plays out. For millions, 'alcoholic' and 'addict' are still terms that make them feel safe. In The Rooms, these words are the equivalent of a secret handshake, a 'Yay, you're with us!' ray of positivity, a language-based emblem.

Outside of The Rooms? I'm not so sure. The evidence tells me otherwise. Witnessing the use of these words myself tells me otherwise. Which is why, nowadays, I've stopped responding to, 'Why aren't you drinking?' (enquires stranger), with the full-beam sunshine bright, 'Because I'm a ragin' alcoholic!' (grin + wink). Which is a shame as it used to be *such fun* to watch them squirm.

To be clear, I've not jettisoned the word altogether. I'll still say I'm an alcoholic if I take someone to a 12-step meeting (if a newbie is meeting-curious) and share, or when talking to fellows of AA, because I know that to say otherwise would be like me saying, 'I'm not with you. I'm not like you.'

When I *am with them, I am like them.* We were all once hopelessly addicted to booze, and now we don't drink any more. Our chosen labels don't change that astronomically powerful shared experience. Any division is unnecessary.

Is it time to pivot?

Overall, given the irrefutable evidence of the stigma around 'alcoholic' and 'addict', which has now been there for 90+ years, I wonder if the experts are right, in that we need a new lexicon. New language with no negativity attached; just as we have created with new adjectives surrounding sexual preference, non-binary gender, race, age, and much more besides.

Society flexes and bends around new descriptors surprisingly nimbly, but the drive for change needs to come from within the sober community themselves. There's no point in health bodies, magazines, rehabs, newspapers and addiction services moving to 'people-first' language if we're continuing to doggedly use 'addiction-as-identity' language.

I've been on national TV and radio dozens of times, talking about recovering from alcohol addiction, and I haven't *once* been introduced as, or labelled as, an 'addict' or 'alcoholic'. Not once! We talked about my past alcohol addiction, my previous raging dependence, without the need for any labels whatsoever. We underestimate society's willingness to change.

I wonder if the lexicon key we are given by others (or snatch up ourselves) as the key to the kingdom, is also the key locking in the stigma (*when it's used in wider society*). Are we unwittingly perpetuating our own stigmatisation by refusing to move with the times? By clinging to tradition?

I wonder if the use of labels such as 'addict' and 'alcoholic' should be reserved for within the community itself, or by invitation only? I don't know what the answer is, but I do know this: we've been trying to shift the stigma for almost 100 years now, by admitting that we're addicts and alcoholics. And the stigma still hasn't shifted. Society at large is already using new language; we're the ones who aren't. Maybe it's now time to finally pivot?

My thoughts on this are not fixed. If I see convincing research that recovery becomes harder without labels, that labels ease recovery, I will flex. Adapt. Recalibrate. And for the record, I would never, ever presume to tell you what to think, or do, or call yourself.

What do you think? Only you can decide.

OUR EXPERTS ON LABELS SUCH AS 'ADDICT' AND 'ALCOHOLIC'

Dr Judith Grisel: 'I think all of the hand-waving around names just confuses. I'm 34 years sober and still call myself a recovering addict. It's helped me take responsibility. And by being "out", I think I may help reduce the stigma. I'm not living under a bridge, as society might expect, I'm a professor and neuroscientist.

At the same time, I do feel like I'm no longer dependent. In the beginning of recovery, I was definitely still dependent, because I was in withdrawal. Now, I'm not.

I've seen it happen. When people say, "I'm an alcoholic" for the first time, it can be really freeing. This is what my problem is. There's something different about my neurobiology that may have pre-existed my using. In my opinion, the label helps remove the blame, but also encourages the taking of responsibility.'

Dr Marc Lewis says: 'The terms "addict" and "alcoholic" are loaded with a fair amount of stigma; it's been that way for decades if not centuries. I sometimes use the term "addict" for brevity and convenience, but I always include a disclaimer that I don't mean it as a put-down, I merely mean it as a classification of an activity, just as I might talk about "students". Many psychiatric diagnostic labels intended to classify people – like "psychotic" – can have all sorts of negative consequences. Whatever a person's issues are, they're not going to fit neatly into any one category. They're a person as a whole.'

Dr David Nutt says: 'I think "alcohol use disorder" is a little overly politically correct. I've never heard anyone say, "I have an alcohol use disorder." Whereas, "I'm an alcoholic" is shorthand in AA for "I'm suffering terribly and need help."

In AA, "alcoholic" and "addict" are mostly used in a positive way, but outside of The Rooms, wider society often uses these words in a negative, stigmatising way. The key is this – labels such as these should never be applied to someone unless they use it first.'

Dr Julia Lewis says: 'When I was a medical student in the 1980s, we were taught not to call people "diabetics" or "asthmatics" any more, given it defines the whole person by the condition. So why are we so incredibly behind with the lexicon around addiction? I use "individual with alcohol dependence" or "with alcohol use disorder". I abhor the terms "alcoholic" and "addict". They carry connotations of blame and self-infliction that we really need to move beyond.'

STONE COLD VS SUNSHINE WARM BIRTHDAYS

STONE COLD DRUNK BIRTHDAY – MY 30TH

'Congrats baby sis!' my brother rejoices, as he pops the champagne with a whoop. I'm squeezed into a storm-grey body-con Hervé Léger dress that I've rented for the night so that I look like the kind of chick who owns designer dresses (I've never owned one in my life).

My dress is fake, my tan is fake, my good mood is fake. There's a micro-shake in my hands as I cheers with my brother and boyfriend. I'm not sure if it's nerves or my need for the alcohol. Both, probably.

I go into my bedroom and privately chug my mood-changer – the rest of the champagne flute. I'm bricking it. Why did I do this? Organise such a huge bash of 50 people? I don't even like big groups of people; they unsettle me. So I'll need more champagne to erode the edges of my fear. I head to the kitchen to recharge my glass, subtly, while my brother and boyfriend chat over their nearly full first glasses.

When we arrive at the venue, the first people I see are frenemies whom I work with. I know they don't like me. I invited them anyway because I really want them to like me.

'Great dress, but your bag looks like it cost about 10p,' says one, flicking her bangle-jangling wrist up and down my body. 'It's ruining everything!' The others laugh.

Great. I'm fooling no one with my rented designer dress and £10 Accessorize diamanté bag.

The cards that mention drinking come thick and fast. I faux-laugh my way through them, while my friends belly laugh. One is more than a little rapey, picturing a face-down woman, her knickers showing beneath her hitched-up dress. It's personalised, for extra shame bang-for-buck.

'Even after 11 wines, Cath was still able to retain her usual ladylike poise.'

Inside, there's a doodle of me, entitled 'BOOZE HAG' (my dubious nickname). The drawing shows a witchy woman with electric-shock hair, clutching a bottle of wine and a cigarette. Nice.

I'm desperately attempting to remain semi-sober (but not too sober; fuck that for a game of soldiers), so that my hippocampus memory-maker doesn't shut up shop for the evening. Why? The blackout hours are the blanks that I fill with the most iniquity. So I ask for a soft drink every other round. It's working. I remember everything up until 1am.

Until the guests begin to straggle away and only the hardcore remain. From then on, I only have ten-second snippets stored, totalling around two minutes remembered from a further two hours.

Fade out. Fade in: there's dancing. Fade out. Fade in: we take a dip in the hot tub. Fade out. Fade in: a taxi home that I fall asleep in.

Most troubling of all is a flashback of me back in my bedroom. I shout at my bewildered boyfriend and tip his laptop onto the floor, like a hellbent kitten with a ball of wool. 'You love your Mac more than me!' is my justification for attempting to trash his most treasured possession. He dives to catch it, like a goalie.

The next morning, he's taking me to Paris. I'm unconscious for our 6am wake-up time. He can't wake me. Scared that I'm going to lash out as I did last night, he enlists the help of my live-in best mate to rouse me. 'Cath, darling,' she gently says, cup of tea proffered in her paw, beatific about being woken at 6am on a Saturday in order to parent me. She's used to it.

I travel to Paris that morning, my first trailblaze through the modern miracle of the Channel Tunnel and my first glimpse of France, with my head on the table, hidden inside my folded arms, desperately trying not to vomit.

The horror only begins to recede once I can legitimately begin drinking again, at lunchtime.

SUNSHINE WARM SOBER BIRTHDAY – MY 40TH

I wake up straight into the security. Up until three years ago, I always woke up into the fear, if only for an infinitesimal split second. 'Where am I? What have I done? What did I drink?'

It's taken my subconscious, the obscured underside of the iceberg in my mind, years to catch up with the fact I no longer have anything to fear. That I no longer wake into wreckages of my own making. In strange beds, strange houses, with strange people.

My boyfriend, sensing somehow that I'm awake (warlock), brings me a coffee. And then he emerges from the kitchen, singing, with a cake, a '4' and '0' ablaze on it. He gives me three small but perfect presents. I open cards. They all say lovely things like, 'We are so proud of you'. There isn't a Booze Hag caricature in sight.

We're in lockdown lite, so a big party is out of the question. But I wouldn't have organised one anyhow, since I know myself better these days. We take a picnic to the Seven Sisters and munch while admiring the view of Beachy Head. The towering 162-metre chalk cliff dwarfs a red-and-white lighthouse. The lighthouse is at least three storeys high but resembles a traffic cone you could kick over.

Powered by cheese, crackers and cake, we hike back to the car, past a field of tiddly Shetland ponies. One shakes his mane and whinnies, all attitude to make up for his diminutive stature. I crop off some emerald-green grass from the verge. 'I have some premium product here for you, sugar,' I say. He pushes his velvety muzzle into my hand. I press my other hand against the star splashed on his forehead. We have a moment.

Later, I meet one of my best mates for a distanced bike ride. She shows up with eight balloons attached to her bike, like a clown. She gives me a badge to pin to my top. 'Awww, how old?' the woman in the shop had asked her while she was buying her birthday wares. 'Er, forty', she'd replied.

We bike until we're underneath the cliffs I was above earlier. Wild purple flowers push their way out of the cliff face, as if demonstrating that grit and grace can dovetail to produce the most unlikely of triumphs.

We stop once we reach Saltdean. There's more cake. This time with a kid's candle shaped like a flower bud. It's meant to bloom open as it plays 'Happy Birthday'. Only, it opens and plays so slowly that it's become creepy, like an off-key jewellery box from a horror film ('whose lock of hair is this?'), or a china doll with a missing eye ('did that doll just move?!').

We find this much funnier than it actually is. The candle is still playing the tinny, sinister ditty ten minutes later, so we have to smash it repeatedly with a rock.

'Happy' – *smash*

'Birth' – *smash*

It emits one final gasp.

'dayyy?' – *SMASH*

The possessed candle is finally dead. And we are crying with laughter.

We ride home, waves pushing their way over the undercliff path, the sun melting into the horizon like a scoop of sorbet on a plate.

I'm in bed by 11pm. There's nothing wild about this birthday whatsoever. Just how I like it.

STONE COLD VS SUNSHINE WARM FESTIVALS

STONE COLD DRUNK FESTIVAL

JULY 2012

Our tomato-red car hums; one of 50 cars serpentine-ing the country roads into the festival. I've been told that Secret Garden Party is like A Midsummer Night's Dream *on acid. Lakes to swim in, glittery fairy people, rope swings, laser shows, abundant trees, gypsy caravans, helter skelters; I can't wait.*

My boyfriend and I swig vodka straight from the bottle, moving approximately six feet every ten minutes. I wear turquoise shorts, a crochet cream top, gladiator sandals and a flowery headband. I'm channelling budget Coachella.

I have a large, purple-dotted wheelie case in the car boot in which I have inexplicably packed nail polish (chips are likely!) and hair straighteners (there might be some sort of beauty airstream with plug outlets!)

I have never camped at a festival before. All I've done are backstage VIP day trips; bonuses that come with my job as a journalist. I have no fucking clue what I'm about to get into.

My boyfriend is more acclimatised, in hiking boots, cargo shorts, a hoodie and a T-shirt with a cartoon dog on it. He has a rucksack in the back. We have vodka, whiskey, rum, beer and cider to keep us going for three nights. It transpires that he's also packed rather a lot of drugs.

'Here, take this,' he says, handing me a tiny blue pill. 'What is it?' 'Diazepam,' he says. 'Like Valium? Am I going to turn into a 1950s housewife who doesn't care that her husband never hoovers?' 'It'll just

chill you out,' he urges. 'Try it.'

I whack it down. Chilling out is very much a desirable. In the past six months my anxiety has entered a hinterland. A hinterland in which the only time I feel calm is three glasses of wine in.

Nowadays, particularly if I'm topping up from the night before, my body and diction seem to get drunk quicker than my brain. I look out from my glassy eyeglobes, a tiny sober person trapped in a drunk person's physicality, as people talk to me slowly and ask if I want water.

'I'm still in here! I'm fine!' I yell, miniature fists beating against my eyeballs, but they don't hear me. They just hear the garble and see the weaving gait.

A peculiar quirk. I'm drinking more these days, but less able to handle it. My tolerance is going down, not up. So I'm already drunk – and Valium-ed – by the time we finally reach the main gate. Damn, I'm relaxed! I feel like when I open the car door, I will slide onto the floor like a pancake person.

I manage to stand, like a regular person. We unpack and I hoist my wheelie case over the wave-peaks of dried mud, defiant as people with backpacks snigger. Worst luck – when we are searched upon entry, patted down in every-which-place but our privates, our belongings upturned – we're told we can't take spirits into the festival. We have to leave the liquor in the car.

But hold up. Maybe this is best luck? As it means I will have unmonitored access to the hardest stuff of all, when I 'go to fetch something' from the car, or 'go to the toilet'. Hmmm. That's good.

We pitch our tent (read: my boyfriend pitches the tent) and head off for a dance with our eight friends. Bella is dressed like a bumblebee. She throws herself around to trance. I just want to have a nap. Sedative upon sedative was perhaps not the wisest.

Over the long weekend, I spend more time in the car park, siphoning off the spirits, trying to psych myself up to go back in, than I do in the *actual festival. I hate the electro, trance, dance, techno music, given I'm an indie chick. I hate our sauna-like tarpaulin crawl space, and I hate what the drugs do to people. The lake does not look appealing for a swim. I can handle drunk people, but here? I see lunatic-eyed nudes crawling around, covered in blue body paint, looking like extras from a schlocky alien B-movie. The toilets are unspeakable.*

My mates offer me 'sharpeners' of cocaine and MDMA, to haul me out of my constant drunk ennui, but all the MDMA does is make me feel sick, and I accidentally tip the coke-taking-mat onto the tarpaulin tent floor. Ten livid eyes swivel to me. 'I need to get out of here,' I slur, getting up and going back to bed for the umpteenth time.

Water is more expensive than alcohol, even if I wanted to buy it. The queue for the shower is longer than that for the bar. And when I try to dance, I no longer have the energy to do it. Sleep is unreachable, unless you're clattered, given our tent is pitched too close to the hardest stage, where the music goes until 3am.

I expected a hedonistic holiday where it is socially permitted to drink from breakfast time – groovy! Everyone's brakes would be off; everyone would be going at it as hard as me. But what I've gotten instead is a neo-apocalyptic Thunderdome in which there is zero chance of recovering from the night before, before going once more unto the breach.

I don't have the wherewithal for any sort of self-care, given I am nearing my final rock bottom. All of my slightly-more-responsible friends, who would normally encourage me to eat, self-care, drink water, wash even, have also torpedoed any notions of self-care. We're all fucked – not just me – this particular weekend. I'm offered ketamine instead of breakfast.

Over three days, I eat a total of two sandwiches and drink maybe two litres of water, maximum. I drink incalculable amounts and take whatever drug I am handed by whatever well-wisher who wants to see me have a 'better time'.

On the way home, caked in mud and humming along in our tomato-red car, I beg my boyfriend to pull over on the motorway lay-by so that I can vomit. 'We're on the twattin' motorway!' he shouts. 'Fuckinhell Cath, you've been a nightmare all weekend. Next time I'm leaving you at home.'

Please do, I think. At least there I'll be warm, dry, clean and able to be alone with wine.

SUNSHINE WARM SOBER FESTIVAL

JULY 2017

I'm at my first sober festival, Boardmasters, aged four. (Years sober, you understand. In earthling years, I am 37).

Boardmasters feels like a semi-wholesome place to cut my teeth, given it's a combination of live music and surfing/skateboarding competitions, set on the curvy Cornish coast. There's a stage called 'The Point', which looks gorgeously incongruous; as if it's been superimposed onto a postcard, given the backdrop of blond sand and crouching cliffs.

It turns out that festivals are fun – and not because of the drinking or the drugs. It turns out that you pick a festival where you want to see the very talented acts on stage, then you see them, and you don't have to configure getting fuckfaced in your arrangement of priorities. Who knew?

I hydrate tactically, so that a one-litre bottle of water lasts me the entire day. I go to the bar once, and the toilet once. I don't need to queue for pints slopping over plastic cups. And then queue again to relieve myself in a diabolical Portaloo. And repeat, for ever. Sober, I spend about 30 minutes of the day in queues, rather than three hours.

I wave at a shellsuit-clad Eighties-style dancer in a rotating cage atop a drinks van. I doubt I'll dance today. My companions aren't fans of dancing, so we'll probably just bob around on the sidelines of the mosh pits.

But then we see The Vaccines. One of my favourite tracks, 'Melody Calling', bursts joyously out of the speakers like a person out of a cake. I can't help myself. I enter the fray and jump around like a lunatic, while my friends look on, nonplussed, shaking their heads, laughing.

I find some teenagers to pogo with. Turns out most teenagers here are not drunk. Did you know that teenagers rarely get drunk these days? Generation Z are already impressing me.

Another surprise; when you're not fixated on spending all of your money on trippin' and getting twatted, the food and shopping opportunities at festivals are splendid. I buy some rad Seventies Levi cut-offs for £7. We dine on chilli and lemon oysters and hunks of freshly baked bread for a tenner. We catch all the acts we want to see and stumble upon some hidden treasures we knew not of.

It's like we've entered an alternative festival dimension that I had no clue existed. Sitting on bales of hay at The Point, listening to a trip-hop band as the clouds suspended over the horseshoe bay turn candyfloss pink, I realise: it's been the perfect day. I've missed out on absolutely nothing by not drinking. I've gained, rather than lost.

The next morning I pound the coral, sunrise-streaked sand, then weave my way around a grassy peninsula where the bushes have been flattened into submission by the wind.

Still panting from my run, I pant past one of tonight's line-up – Jay Kay from Jamiroquai – having breakfast on a hotel terrace. Wearing a huge hat before 9am, he's clearly a method frontman. The rest of his band come back from the buffet with their thimbles o' juice and tiny croissants, all also wearing daft headgear. I smile at them.

I love festivals.

IS ALCOHOL A PARENTING AID?

I'm not a parent but I've received thousands of drinking stories from those who are. What's struck me is this: there's often an expectation that becoming a parent will tame or slow the drinking. The reality is: becoming a parent can accelerate it. I've been told that, as beautiful as the experience is, it's also when the shit hits the fan (sometimes literally) and, thus, it can make a growing dependence dig its claws in harder.

Heavy drinking + parenting is riotously enabled by society. I walked through the supermarket today and saw a babygro chirruping 'I'm why Daddy drinks' and a book called *Why Mummy's Sloshed*. And then I saw that *Workin' Moms* had just dropped on Netflix, illustrated by a still life of a baby bottle and a wine bottle. 'Wine on the lips, baby on the hips' marketing is now unbelievably omnipresent. I'm told this was not the case a decade or so ago; parents were not constantly told they needed alcohol to parent. Now, they are.

How does this 'alcohol is a parenting aid!' messaging affect actual parents? I asked them.

'Apparently my non-drinking ruined her son's birthday party'

Harper says: 'I was at a four-year-old's birthday party when it happened. I said "no thanks" to a wine and had a whole tableful of mums chanting at me: "HAVE A WINE! HAVE A WINE! HAVE A WINE!" It was kinda funny, but also it wasn't, because I was only a few weeks sober and I'd been honest with them as to why I wasn't drinking. I told them it made me anxious and hangovers meant I didn't want to do anything with the kids. Then I was told by the host that I was ruining her son's birthday by not drinking. I waited for the chanting to die down and then went off to do some Lego with the kids. I'm over a year sober now. Funny thing: the more people try to make me drink now, the more I don't want to. It awakens the rebel in me. When I was 13 I rebelled by hanging around the shop and waiting for an adult willing to buy us alcohol. Now, I'm rebelling by not drinking.'

'My post-birth recovery plan was daily wine'

Stella says: 'I wasn't able to breastfeed my son, which broke my heart, but was also a massive relief – it meant I could drink. I declared that my post-birth recovery plan was wine, and that I intended to drink wine daily for six weeks after my C-section. Given we were brought champagne as gifts, it made total sense.

I drank roughly a bottle of wine a night. I now understand that I had post-natal depression for the first six months. Although the drinking seemed celebratory on the surface, I think I was trying to find relief from the exhaustion and adrenaline.

Of course, while drinking, I had social media, memes and mothers on TV on my side. My husband's a nurse who does long shifts, so alcohol seemed like the perfect parenting aid. It gave me company, comfort and connection, or so I thought. I turned up to a first birthday party with a bottle of wine, and my friend said, "We're not going to drink this now, is that OK? Are you OK? You seem detached." I was in a total fog, because of the PND.

It took me until my son was three to realise there was an issue, and he was five when I stopped. I'm coming up on 18 months sober. In hindsight, I wish I'd told my GP the truth, or at least an approximation of the truth. But I didn't want to be told to stop. Club Soda on socials helped me hugely. I posted every day for a year. I'll teach my son that drinking is not a default position. It's valid to want to *not* drink.'

'We do the marketing for them when we cheers to "wine o'clock" with our "mummy juice".'

Alexis says: 'It's 4.30am. I've been up since 2am. So far, reasons for this include my youngest daughter (who is autistic and has learning difficulties) wanting milk, needing a wee, wanting to watch *Shaun the Sheep*, asking me to let her teacher know she ate jam on toast for the first time, insisting she is going to wear her black coat tomorrow, wanting more milk (resulting in a small battle when I say no), needing another wee and demanding to have a bath (resulting in a big battle when I say no), and then me giving in and letting her watch *Shaun the Sheep*. CHEERS SHAUN.

I am fucking tired.

Big Alcohol tells parents (mainly mums) that because parenting is challenging, we deserve wine and gin. It pushes this ridiculous, irresponsible and dangerous messaging on us and, even worse, we push it on ourselves. We do the marketing for them when we cheers to "wine o'clock" with our "mummy juice".

If I'd drunk last night, I would have felt horrendous having been up since 2am. I would have been impatient and snappy. It's my privilege (not job) to be the one my daughter needs right now. I don't "deserve" alcohol for the tough days, but I do deserve to take it easy, catch up on sleep and maybe order a takeaway.

To be really clear, I'm not making judgements about parents who drink. I'm calling bullshit on the irresponsible media messaging that asserts wine is an essential tool for parenting. I can't think of any parenting scenario that would be improved by alcohol. Not one. Not even kids' birthday parties, which I think should be up there with weddings as sober "firsts" in terms of milestones.

Talking of which, when my eldest (now 15) was young, there was no booze at kids' birthday parties. With my youngest (now six), it's at every party. It's normal that you bring a present *and* a bottle. I think it's used as a social lubricant to ease the awkwardness. It's all small talk, people comparing their kids and outlining what they eat for dinner. Nowadays, unless it's a friend's kid, I ask if I can drop off, rather than stay at the party.

Our kids are seeing this. Water bottles with boozy slogans implying it's gin, paper cups filled with wine. What are we teaching them about coping mechanisms? "Hard day at school, have a glass of wine"? "Got an exam, have a wine!"

I quit drinking when my eldest was 12. There was a time when she was my wine waitress at dinner parties. Then I got sober, and that's influenced her attitude to alcohol. She's never tried drinking (aged 15) and says she doesn't even want it at her future wedding.

As for parenting with a hangover? That absolutely sucks. I remember changing a nappy and throwing up while I was doing it. Do you want a picture of me doing that on social media?'

'We put bottles of wine under pushchairs to drink in the park.'

Laura says: 'Nearly four years ago my husband and I adopted two little girls, aged two and four. The early life trauma they suffered has affected their judgement of the world, so parenting them can be pretty tough. My husband and I opened a bottle of wine every night to debrief. For the first 18 months of parenting, we drank every night. Come the summer, we'd sit in the garden so we could start drinking in the afternoon: prosecco with a frozen raspberry. During a lot of those nights, we were merry when the girls went to bed, and then we'd continue drinking. I felt guilty at weekends because I was hungover and couldn't do as much with the girls as I wanted to.

Pair that with my new "mummy friends" and trouble was brewing. We'd meet up for coffee mornings where more buck's fizz was drank than coffee. We started a book club; merely a ploy to drink more often together. A running club ended up in the pub. There were times we met after school with bottles of wine under the pushchair, to drink in the park. Servings of wine in paper cups with stripey straws at 3pm. Our Facebook page featured memes about goldfish bowl glasses of gin.

My last drink was at a mum friend's summer BBQ. I was the first to leave, at 10pm. I got up the next morning, but spent the afternoon on the sofa with a stonking headache. "Mummy, what are we doing now?" I felt awful that I couldn't play with them.

My mum friends know I don't drink now. But on my last birthday, one gave me a bottle of prosecco regardless, "Because I thought you might like to drink at some point." Weird.

I love that, now, my girls see me having a restful weekend rather than being unable to get my butt up out of the chair because I'm feeling ropey. I sleep better and wake up fresh. I love that they see me go running and bouncing back to make a healthy breakfast. They're six and eight now. I don't feel the need to have something to make me *more* relaxed now – because I *am* more relaxed.'

'I became sober-curious at the same time my teens became alcohol-curious.'

Freddie says: 'After kids, I started drinking at home in a way I never had before. My kids are now 15 and 17 and I quit on my 50th birthday. Before that, I felt enormous shame about my kids saying to me, "You're drunk", when I lost my patience with them. I've fallen over in front of them. And my son Tom's propped me up before, walking home from a night out.

I became sober-curious at the same time they became alcohol-curious. They now both drink, even though they're not of legal age. Alcohol is pushed absolutely everywhere, and I've seen this steadily increase in the past 15–20 years, so I really want to show my kids that they don't need alcohol to grow into themselves.

I'm open with them about scrapes I got into, which wouldn't have happened if I wasn't drunk. In turn, Tom is confiding in me. In a fit of jealousy, he recently punched a fence and told me that he felt like getting into a car to drive, but didn't. I'm glad he can tell me these things.

My sister and I were parented by my father because my mum had a mental-health condition and was dependent on alcohol. She'd be in bed all day, then get up in the evening and drink. We talked a lot about my mum's mental-health issues, but never alcohol. This strikes me as strange now, but maybe it's a generational thing, in that he didn't know how to talk about it.

Nobody said to me at that age: "you don't have to drink". Nobody told me it was normal to feel uncomfortable in my own skin as a teen. So now I impart these messages to my kids.

It used to really piss me off on a Friday night if I needed to stay sober just in case my kids needed me to drive them. These days, I tell them that if they need picking up in the middle of the night, I'm there. And now I'm sober, I can be.'

'MAYBE YOU CAN MODERATE NOW?' SAYS THE VOICE

I will make a bold statement now. I'd wager that 99 per cent of sober stalls, slips, relapses, whatever you want to call them, are down to the 'maybe now it will be different? Maybe now we can moderate?' voice. Which, in my mind, emits from a tiny, obsessed Gollum sat on my shoulder.

Thankfully, these days, my waking 'moderate?' Gollum is totally silent. My rational, awake-hours brain knows, beyond the shadow of a doubt, that given I attempted moderation on roughly 3,276 occasions over 21 years ('That was you trying to moderate?!' said one friend, in utter disbelief. *Yes really,* that was me trying to moderate) and only successfully moderated on perhaps 30 of those (if that!), moderation ain't ever gonna happen for me. Nor would I want it to, given I have no conscious notion of wanting a drink these days.

Even so, every six months or so, my subconscious will try to persuade me, via the fantasia of a dream, that moderation is now within reach or, indeed, desirable. During the pandemic, I had this dream. I was on a plane (already unlikely scenario, in lockdown) and ordered two tiny bottles of wine (likely scenario, when I was boozing) and then after those... I stopped drinking (wildly unlikely scenario). Basically, when I'm asleep, that's when my subconscious gets a chance to run around inside my brain and present this airplane scenario where I can moderate.

I'm ultra-gullible, but even I know that's bullshit.

Let me tell you a story to illustrate how *infamous* I am for being gullible. Here's a conversation I had last night while seated at a bar.

***

Him: 'Don't look now, but there's a clown behind you.'

I start to turn around. He places a hand on my arm.

Him: 'Don't! It's rude. It looks a bit pissed off. And it's looking straight at us.'

Me: 'Seriously? What kind of clown?'

Him: 'A circus one.'

Me: 'Is it alone?'

Him: 'Seems to be. It has some balloons.'

At this point I am feeling almost tearful – who likes pissed-off clowns boring eyeholes into their back? But he has doubled over with laughter.

I smell a rat.

I turn.

No clown.

Yup. Gullible.

***

Nonetheless, that same night, as we watched the smokin' and squat, salt-crowned and curvy, globe-glassed and sorbet-bright cocktails sail past us – high above the crowd on trays – there's one thing I'll never, ever believe. A voice inside me – or outside of me, or in a dream – saying, 'Hey! I think it'll be different this time! This 3,277th time.' Because no, voice, people or dream; it won't be. I don't believe you.

I'll believe you if you tell me there's a pissed-off clown behind me, but on this point? Not buying it.

II: YEAR SIX

YEAR SIX: WE REPEAT WHAT WE DON'T REPAIR

In year six, I finally feel ready to deep-dive into uncharted leagues. My childhood. I've skated on the surface of those fathoms but I haven't immersed and explored. When I do, it proves to be both arduous and illuminating, beastly and beautiful.

Strong statement coming atcha: I think that untangling your childhood in therapy is one of the most important things to do, if not *the most*, in order to bloom into long-term recovery.

Why? Because having a tough time in childhood means you are seven times more likely to become addicted to alcohol later in life. This makes childhood trauma THE chart-topping predisposition to addiction. Above any other factor, hands down. It's the singular, sole, top predictor.

We know this because from 1995 to 1997 the CDC and Kaiser Permanente performed a massive study on 17,000 Americans. They found that four or more ACEs (an ironic misnomer of an acronym, given ACE stands for Adverse Childhood Experiences) denotes the sevenfold 'later addiction' prophecy.

'It's a very high correlation,' confirms Dr Marc Lewis. 'As a psychotherapist, I'd say that almost everyone I treat with addiction problems – 90 per cent – has had real difficulties in childhood or adolescent years.' He pauses and then adds. 'In fact, it's probably 100 per cent.'

When we talk of ACEs, we're not talking about isolated events. 'It's very hard to raise a kid perfectly,' Dr Marc Lewis acknowledges. 'But we're not talking about just sloppy parenting here; we're talking shaming, painful and sometimes abusive experiences.'

Traumatised, me? Nah

Let's backtrack, for a moment, to the term 'childhood trauma'. Trauma is a strong word, right? For me, a 'traumatic childhood' summons images from *War Child* campaigns. Of a brutal existence under a leaky tin roof, of no shoes, of war-torn conflict, kids holding rifles, and shanty towns.

And, of course, that is a savage reality for many. So how dare we in the West, most of whom have been sheltered, shod and fed our entire lives, lay claim to the term 'trauma'? Oh no, did your Daddy not buy you a pony? Did Mummy not plait your hair? Did your folks not make you three-course meals? How terribly frightful!

To cry trauma feels like perverted first-world privilege: my feather pillow was too soft, my toy-filled room was too warm, my Game Boy was too bright. And yet, even if you had all of the trappings of the Western world, you can still suffer from post-childhood trauma.

'Adverse Childhood Experiences are *so* prevalent and not the reserve of children in war zones,' says psychologist and neuroscientist Dr Judith Grisel. 'An ACE can be as simple as economic stress or witnessing parents fight.'

'I think the rise in alcohol addiction is definitely linked to the rise of early trauma,' adds Dr Grisel. But with a nuance. She thinks the ACEs and early drinking are dominoes. 'The ACEs are a proxy for early drinking. It's the kids experiencing ACEs who don't sit down to dinner with parents, who are unsupervised, who are given too much freedom and thus pick up too young,' she says. Which then dominoes into dependence. *ACEs – early use – addiction* go the dominoes. (We'll come back to early drinking in a later chapter, don't worry)

You'll likely be surprised to learn what counts as an ACE. I was.

Regularly being sworn at, insulted or humiliated counts as one ACE. As does having felt your family was not supportive or close. Any sexual contact whatsoever with someone five or more years older. Violence against your mother. Or living with an adult who was then addicted or mentally ill.

'Pain changes – it develops and evolves,' says Dr Marc Lewis. 'What starts as insecurity, frustration and confusion in childhood might translate into anger, depression, addiction, eating disorders, OCD, so on. The origins hold the pain in place and act as a causal springboard.'

At the bottom of this page,* there's a link to a questionnaire where you can figure out your ACE score. Remember: four or more ACEs means you were seven times more predisposed to alcohol addiction *before you even started drinking*. Go and have a look-see, if you're curious. I was shocked at my score; you may well be too.

***

Of course, a one-page questionnaire can't cover every nuance of childhood neglect or upset.

- It's the kid subject to pageant parenting, wheeled out as a life-size doll. Who feels held hostage by a ~~Tiger~~ Peacock Mother. Whose natural zitty, smelly, hairy, curvy adolescence is treated as anathema. Not a hair out of place, please darling.

- It's the latchkey kid ignored as soon as they can reach all of the kitchen appliances, who became a mini-adult, in charge of microwaving their own beige meals.

---

* https://tinyurl.com/y3hmoc28
If for any reason this link doesn't work, go to https://www.ncjfcj.org and search for 'Finding your ACE score'.

- It's the teenager who lies in bed above a domestic war zone. Who listens to muffled expletives, jumps at mysterious bangs, turns over and tries to sleep while their heart is galloping. In the morning, they tiptoe downstairs and clear up broken glass from drunken rows.

- It's the child made responsible for their parents' feelings, in the topsy-turvy phenomenon 'parentification'. Who is given the dubious honour of being their parents' main source of comfort, when it ought to be the other way around.

- Or in a supersized version of that, it's the child made aware of the suicidal ideation of the parent. Who lives on tenterhooks, who becomes *the parent*. Who watches like a hawk for darkening moods.

- It's the child become confidante, who is used as a pawn against the other parent, in that they know way too much about infidelities, domestic violence, or transgressions within their parents' broken marriage. A child is not meant to know about such adult themes – or indeed, be a parent's best friend.

- It's the child told they were unwanted, a mistake, or more baldly, that their parents wish they'd never been born. Who grows up believing they owe an eternal debt, merely for having been conceived.

- The teen whose privacy is invaded by the almost inaudible soft click that means someone else has picked up a linked house phone. Whose diaries are invaded. Who's punished for the contents of these private conversations and thoughts.

- The child who's smacked and slapped. When they raise this in adulthood they're told 'It never did you any harm!' But in today's enlightened world, we can see the undeniable harm caused by a child being thwacked across the face by someone twice their size.

- It's the teen whose every expressed emotion is batted away as them being 'too sensitive' or 'melodramatic'; and who, therefore, learns to stuff down and ignore their wants and needs. Taught from year dot to disconnect from their desires, and to instead hitch their wagon to the star of *other people's desires*. They become classic people-pleasers, growing in resentment as every year rolls by in which they don't serve their own needs.

Childhood trauma is often much more subtle than the abuse that would cause social services to swoop in: it's often harsh words rather than beatings with a belt; it's a house full of food but empty of love; it's eggshells on the kitchen floor and unreasonable levels of chores. It's conditional love.

The puncture wound that ACEs leave is how addiction gets in. Addiction burrows into that pinprick of childish tragedy, of soft-skinned injury. Which is why it's so imperative that in long-term recovery, we learn to find that wound and treat it as best we can. Otherwise, that toy-proportioned trauma will never fully give us peace. We may even go on to recreate the dysfunctional households we were raised in. In the words of therapist Christine Langley-Obaugh: 'We repeat what we do not repair.'

Early stress shapes us like Play-Doh

My childhood was, like most, a smushed-up mixture of heaven and hell. It was bad–good. Good–bad.

Up until the age of nine, I am pretty happy. I'm well-liked at school and have a best friend called Jane. I like playing kerby and nicking my brother's BMX; I like making daisy chains and writing to the Care Bears via the magical Post Office portal of the underside of my pillow (the Care Bears are my mother, it turns out).

We live in a cul-de-sac in Carrickfergus, where the kids can play safely unsupervised (although we live in primal fear of the dog that bit Connor's bum, a source of suburban legend). I recall hazy days sitting under a fuchsia bush, my first crush, being teacher's pet, trips to my grandparents' sweet shop, cheese on toast and my Grandpa Smurf.

Then my parents get divorced. Which is not necessarily a bad thing in and of itself, since a child raised in an increasingly embittered home is likely just as affected as a child raised in a split home. But it sets off a chain of events.

Our house is sold. My mother, brother and I move to Belfast for a spell – and then we move on to England when I'm ten. My Dad stays in Northern Ireland, as do all my friends and family. The England move is the very opposite of what I want. But I must confess I'm impressed by the police stations that look like cottages rather than Fort Knox; that have flower boxes rather than barbed wire.

I struggle to fit into my new school and have a strong Northern Irish accent. Alas, we don't say 'here' when roll call is read, or waggle our hands in the air, we are assigned a number, and my number – 28 – is probably the least kind number for a NI child trying to blend into an English school. My classmates cruelly mimic my 'Twennyaahate'.

I'm frequently asked if my dad is a 'bomber' or in the IRA. I'm not popular. In fact, I have my first fight in the playground, a stand-off of slaps, when I attempt to clear my dad's name. I start having nightmares about the kids at school creeping into our garden and climbing up the drainpipe.

Time for high school. We're moving house again. To Dudley this time, as my mother has met her soon-to-be second husband. We move to a large, lovely house with a big garden next to a park: a serious upgrade from our tiny terrace. Signs point to sunshine.

However, it turns out my new stepfather openly hates us. His child, who visits intermittently, is called 'treasure' while my brother and I are called 'the lodgers'. We are told we are moving out the instant we turn 18. I count the years back on my chubby child hands.

At 12, I start drinking.

We are not allowed in the living room past 7pm, whereupon we are banished to our rooms. Friends who dare to call on me spontaneously are sent away with a roar and a slam, so they stop calling. My stepfather reads my diaries. Even my phone calls are listened to.

At 13, I start clubbing with older friends.

We receive typed letters from our stepfather about how we are contravening our lodging agreement. Too much butter left on knives in the dishwasher! Making a noise with the Hoover doing our chores while he is trying to write the next *Lord of the Rings*!

At 14, I start experimenting with drugs.

And finally, he chases me around the house when I'm 15, for eating some of his pork pie. 'I should have beaten you up long ago!' he yells. I tear my way up to my brother's room and hide behind his bed. My brother blocks my stepfather's path to me. My mum then kicks him out. But we've spent four formative years under his despotic rule.

Meanwhile, on parallel-story tracks; when I'm 11, my father who is still in Northern Ireland, meets a lovely woman called Ruth. She becomes my 'second mum'. Our thrice-yearly trips there are the happiest days of my childhood. Treasure hunts, joyful Christmases, trips to the beach with Jack Russells, Coke floats, frisbee wars, Donegal caravan holidays with Swingball and exhilarating swims in the lough.

Aged 12, I ask my dad if I can move in with him and Ruth. I beg, in fact. Ruth says yes, he says no. I am devastated. They later split when I'm 15. I start dividing my holidays between my two parents in Northern Ireland; my biological parent in Belfast (my dad) and my logical parent on Islandmagee (Ruth).

Back in England: when I'm 16, we move again. I move in with my new stepfather and stepfamily before my mother does, so that I can start sixth form. We've lucked out this time; my new stepfather is the kindest man I've ever met. His family too.

But my social anxiety is now so shrill that making friends at the new sixth form is challenging. The common room, full of insouciant tangled teenage limbs, is about as welcoming as a bear pit. I fall in with a crowd of art-room stoners who spend lunchtime in the woods, drinking. Socialising without alcohol is becoming unthinkable, although at this point, I'm still also a mega-nerd (I hand in extra essays, which my English teacher looks at like, '*thannnnks*', as if she hasn't got enough marking to do).

A few years from now, Ruth will be diagnosed with breast cancer for the second time at 45. I spend her last Christmas with her, watching her be eaten from the inside out by cancer. I'm devastated.

And so, that's you up to speed. I'm sure you've already guessed that this is not my *whole* story; it's the 'safe for work' version of my childhood. It's had the gnarliest parts cut, for my and others' sanity.

Nonetheless, even the uncut-for-public version isn't particularly remarkable or tragic. Divorce, much moving, wicked/wonderful stepparents, privacy invasion, threats of physical abuse and losing a (logical) parent, are not all that uncommon. And yet my ACE score was six. Which places me well into the sevenfold prophecy zone. What about you? What's your score?

Addiction as a seized second childhood

A stress-studded childhood often has a paradoxical effect. It means you grow up *much* too fast but simultaneously stay frozen in partial arrested development, having never grown up properly at all. Our developments both speed up and stall. What a curious contradiction.

Toddlers are constantly compared to tiny drunkards – '7 reasons babies are just tiny drunk adults' has over two million views on YouTube. 'They fall asleep everywhere', 'The munchies' and 'They can't hide their feelings' are a few of the seven reasons. It's straight-up hilarious, featuring toddlers falling asleep in cakes, snogging mirrors and pulling out an entire shelf of a fridge in a bid to get a snack.

So yes. There are many parallels. But it's not actually toddlers behaving like drunk adults. Think about it. That makes no sense. It's more that drunk adults have devolved to become their previous toddler selves.

I was struck by this revelation recently, watching a toddler call her parent a 'bumhead' for taking her juice shoot off her, and being reminded that I once called my boyfriend an 'arsehole' for taking my cider off me. A toddler lying down in the supermarket because they can't have a Paw Patrol magazine? I once lay down in a road because I wanted to get a taxi rather than the night bus.

When drunk, it's somehow socially permitted to behave like a toddler. People *do* tell us the next day what nightmares we were, but if we were sober when we put in performances like that, the talking-to would be much more stern.

I wonder whether heavy drinking is a roundabout way of seizing that which we often skipped some of. Having a second childhood of sorts. Is it a way of our dissatisfied inner child snatching a slice of childhood that they felt robbed of first time around?

Recovery is also infantile, in many ways. Those in rehab are parented; literally given chores and told when/what to eat. Outside of rehab, we move back home, or take time out of work. We need a childlike existence to bounce back. It's why I returned to the nest *and* watched an indecent amount of Pixar films in very early recovery.

Often we have to go backwards in order to actually launch this time, rather than faux-launch by swaggering out a guesstimation of what we think an adult ought to look like. We go back to re-learn how to look after ourselves, how to get enough sleep, nourish ourselves, medicate stress without merlot, and not hose-spray all of our money away, like an F1 driver with a bottle of champagne.

In recovery, we finally grow up. But to do that fully, we have to go back. Not just physically; emotionally too.

The work begins

And so I do. I start weekly therapy*, with someone who has ample experience with digging around in ACEs. I develop an almost pathological mania for reading about, learning about, how our childhoods impact our adult lives.

I read *The Body Keeps the Score* by Bessel van der Kolk and discover that we literally hold traumatic childhood experiences in

---

* Many therapists and counsellors do means-tested fees, meaning you can sometimes get sessions for a discount. At the time of writing, Brits can refer themselves for free talking therapy via the NHS without even having to go through their GP. Search for 'IAPT' services on www.nhs.uk.

our bodies. I devour School of Life book *How to Overcome your Childhood*, which triggers mind revolutions with practically every turn of the page. I pick it up half-heartedly at 11pm and find myself spellbound until 3am. Upon which I buy three copies for friends, in the hope they might feel the same tectonic shift within.

Those laden with ACEs are like rescue dogs. But unlike the often mysterious back-history of rescue dogs, we have the privilege of knowing about our own pock-marked lineage. We know where it hurts. Luckily, simply knowing where to go is half of the battle.

Echoes and connections

As if spellbound by a gypsy curse, it's ACE recovery 101 that many of us unconsciously recreate undesirable childhoods.

- The kid who was treated badly by their parents often grows up to treat themselves badly too. And maybe others also.

- The child whose parents shouted and swore will likely gravitate towards romantic partners who shout and swear.

- The children who grew up watching their parents drink themselves to oblivion, or smoke themselves silly, will loathe it at the time, but often later mimic that behaviour.

It's horribly unfair and we don't even realise we're doing it. We just re-enact the familiar, even if the familiar was fearsome. Being aware of it, and consciously changing the echo, is the one and only imperative antidote to the curse.

I learn that trauma is like a vast electrical network. That a surge from someplace that seems very far away, unrelated, can trigger a rise in us all the way over here. That what happened when we were four can still short-circuit our behaviour when we are forty.

I start paying close attention to my impulses, behaviours, irrational reactions, illogical thought loops. I discover that things that seem entirely unconnected are connected. My urge to spring-clean my flat, for instance, when I feel like I'm in trouble, is related to something specific. I trace a silvery wire leading from the 40-year-old me back to the 11-year-old me.

I gain the ability to step back and see patterns, whereas before I was just caught in a chaotic clusterfuck where something would spark me off, yet I didn't know why. Once you know *why* something makes you overreact, or hurts you disproportionately, or indeed has you disinfecting the cutlery drawer, you can start to apply adult tools to a childlike tripped fuse.

Empaths: the canaries in the coalmine

I don't know I'm an empath until my therapist tells me I am.

'It's like I can catch people's feelings,' I say.

'How so?' she asks.

'Like if I'm sat next to someone on a train and they're stressed. I start to feel stressed too. It's like they carry a cloud that I get sucked into.'

'Do you feel that with loved ones too, as well as strangers?'

'With loved ones it's even more potent. If someone I love is upset and I'm near them, I can't detach from their emotion. It's like they're carrying an aura and I get lost in it too. Even if I walked into the house feeling sunflower-yellow, I wind up feeling storm-grey, if they are.'

'You may be an empath,' she says.

An empath is someone who absorbs others' emotions. Feels

their joy, pain, stress, sorrow. Those with tumultuous childhoods often become empaths because it was an enormously useful skill as a little, to be able to read the emotions of the bigs. It kept us safe and in favour, to not only have our wits about us, but have them sharpened.

A 2018 study showed that those who've experienced trauma in childhood demonstrate 'elevated empathy' as adults when compared to those who had a peachy childhood. In a *specific* type of empathy, though. 'Affective empathy', which the study defines as 'the ability to respond to another person's mental state with an appropriate emotion'. Cognitive empathy, or 'the ability to understand another's thoughts and feelings', was not higher in those with ACEs.

This means that empaths are not necessarily supreme beings when it comes to placing ourselves in another's shoes, or at intellectualising why another might feel that way; but we are excellent at mirroring and thus 'catching' another's emotion.

It's a blessing *and* a curse, of course. Being a human antenna for joy is pretty handy, or being able to feel and share in someone's excitement. Poet Kahlil Gibran once wrote, 'The deeper that sorrow carves into your being, the more joy you can contain.' Which is a beautiful truth. But it's when we're catching – containing – micro-aggression, worry, irritation or depression that empaths suffer.

Of course, sometimes you want to feel an emotion in tandem with a loved one. To twin with their grief, or frustration, or anger, in order to help them through it. But if we find ourselves consistently absorbing other's negative states when we don't want or need to (our co-workers for instance, or strangers), there are ways to become less permeable.

Here's my trick. I'll be in my co-working space sitting next to someone deep-sighing and tutting with stress. GREAT, I'll think. Here we go. Here it comes. And I'll allow it in at first. Let it peak, like a wave. Allowing it in allows it to wash through me. It then recedes, as a tide would recede. It's coming back, though. But this time I'm imagining a bubble around me; almost like a zorb ball. And so, instead of getting soaked to the skin, I can bob around on the surface and dry off.

If I'm going into a situation with a loved one where I know there will be ample negativity, I now already have my zorb ball on. At first, this felt like betrayal, or being insensitive, or uncaring. But now I know that it's just good mental health. We don't have to be walking containers for the emotions of others, like a water drum on legs. We can practise our 'cognitive empathy' skills rather than being beholden to 'affective empathy', which simply pours another's emotions into us, whether we like it or not.

Who's mad at me today?

Alongside 'affective empathy', another offshoot of an ACE-strewn childhood is 'abject paranoia' (not a clinical term, I just made it up).

A *New Yorker* cartoon (by Brendan Loper and Ellis Rosen) recently made me squeak, in the manner of a stepped-on pet toy. It's entitled 'Who's mad at me?' and depicts a bloke staring at what looks like a pictorial family tree. He strokes his chin, musing, as he looks at each loved one's face. 'Emi?', 'Ben?', 'Sam?'

It perfectly sums up what goes on in my head, regularly. On a fortnightly basis I experience 'abject paranoia' that a family member is falling out of love with me. An unreturned email can send me spiralling into a constellation of paranoia in which I feel adrift in a zero-gravity blank space where their reply should be. I tell myself stories as to why they might be mad at me. I imagine our relationship breaking down. I script what they'll say, and what I'll say. I even dream about it. It's *so relaxing*.

And then I see them, or they return my email, or we talk, and I find out that everything's fine. Of course it is. They were just busy, or rushed, or have other things going on that I knew not of.

I have delivered sincere apologies such as, 'I'm so sorry I didn't give you more attention when you sprained your ankle', because a contact lull has led me to spin a doom-laden tale whereby they are fucked off with me because of sprained-ankle neglect. I received the reply, 'What are you on about, you big banana?!'

And so, all is well. I feel a brief spell of cosy warmth... and then I find someone else to be neurotic about. *Oh, what about them, though? Maybe they're mad at me? Probably.* It's a self-loathing and narcissism orgy, but with a bowlful of ACE-laced steroids instead of keys.

It turns out your regular person doesn't do this. Did you know that? I didn't. They don't constantly hunt people's faces for clues of failing love, or imagine familial connections doing a midnight flit, or think a text without a kiss on it means the Ice Age has begun.

I learn through therapy that this is common when we've been taught somewhere along the way, by *someone* (whoever it may be), that familial love is conditional, withdrawable, inconstant and dependent on you being a 'good person.'

Now that I know this, I can trace the 'Who's mad at me?' wire to that teaching, take a long hard look at it and chuck the misbegotten belief into the bin. The belief then makes its way back, like an enchanted object. So over and over I have to do it.

Nine times out of ten, even if they were indeed 'mad' at you, that cannot torpedo family love. Which is usually unconditional, no matter how much of a raging twit you are. It's something that can withstand knocks, awkwardness, an unexplained freeze-over and an inexplicable thaw. Love ebbs and flows, yes, but it's always *there*. And it's not dependent on a tit-for-tat, given vs owed, transactional exchange.

If it's not always there, if it *truly is conditional*, then that's for the conditional love-giver to hold, not us. If you look at their other relationships, you'll find this pattern repeats itself, which makes it feel less intensely personal. They're like that with everyone. Not just wretched, rejected, frozen-out us. It's a revelation, to realise.

Buttons

If something makes you react in a disproportionate way, it's likely you have what I like to call 'a button' there. Michael A. Singer, author of *The Untethered Soul*, calls these 'thorns' and encourages us to relax into them. Buddhists tend to call them wounds – advocating dharmic detachment. Soberland uses 'trigger' and advises a focus on the only thing you *can* control – your reaction. Keeping your side of the street clean. *Their* side is their business.

All my reading and therapy leads me to do something unprecedented. I make a map of my buttons. I name them all. My buttons are: feeling judged/criticised (pretty universal one this), feeling told what to do/think (I ardently believe people should do/think what they want, but I can't control others) and feeling taken advantage of (especially in terms of unfair work division).

Then there's being rushed (people showing up early/chasing me if they're early), not being 'allowed' enough alone/quiet time (this is why audible texting taps/buzzes/bleeps on phones in public do my head in) and feeling manipulated or guilt-tripped ('you are only a good person if you...' or 'if you loved me, you would...')

What's more, I now know where all of these buttons originate; what their power source is. And so when someone presses one, or two in tandem, I know why their action or comment bothers me. Rather than just allowing the button press to send me Buckarooing in response, or allowing it to emit a rote response from me, like a talking bear, I can then choose how to respond.

These buttons get pushed all the time, but that doesn't mean it's <insert person> to blame. *C'est la vie*, baby. Monitoring them is ultimately my responsibility. My reaction is on me.

I am not a toy. I have buttons, but I choose what to do when they are pushed. You are not a toy either. We are people and we choose our reactions, no matter what the button-presser's action or comment was. As sentient beings, rather than talking bears, we have what I like to call 'the gift of the golden pause'.

What are your buttons? If we name them, make a map of them and draw links back to where they originated, we can gain more power over them. Our backflip bucks and automated responses may well become less likely.

Backpack of rocks

TRIGGER WARNING: Experiences of childhood sexual abuse discussed (pages 140–2).

Many of us go into adulthood carrying a rock or two. Maybe even a backpack of rocks. We can go through our entire lives without unpacking these rocks. The rocks are episodes in our childhood when we were sexualised by adults.

I won't tell you about my rocks. A person, even one who writes so publicly about the personal and believes fiercely in the healing power of doing so, has to keep some things private. Because revealing

---

* Brits who have experienced traumatic childhoods can access free support groups via www.napac.org.uk.

all? Therein madness lies. But I will tell you about my pebble.

I'm around 10. I'm being babysat by a man with a beard. I know him. I feel comfortable with him. My brother is in bed. Bearded Man has let me stay up late, but has sent my brother to bed. In your face, brother! I win.

Bearded Man has put on a film about Adam and Eve. They're naked in it, ooheee! It's certified as a 15 film. I know it's naughty that I'm watching this. My tiny body is taut about the transgression of seeing adult nipples and bottoms.

Nonetheless, when Bearded Man suggests we take our clothes off like Adam and Eve, my thrill shuts down. *No*, I say. *I don't want to*, I say. I move away from him. He drops it. He doesn't push it. But I'll never forget that scene and that feeling, of an adult male's eyes roaming over my body for the first time.

I didn't tell anyone. Why? Bearded Man set my silence up carefully, by making me promise I wouldn't tell anyone, as he slid the VHS into the player. 'I'll get into trouble for letting you watch a 15 film,' he said. 'So this has to be our secret. Do you swear?' he added. I nodded my ringlet-covered head solemnly, crossed my heart and hoped to die, intoxicated by the notion of watching a 15. The glamour!

Therefore, I thought disclosure of the peculiar incident of the 15 film in the night-time ('Daddy, so-and-so suggested we take our clothes off last night') would get us both into trouble, so I didn't tell. I wasn't a snitch, after all. My little head filed it under '15 film fun! No big deal' especially because I wasn't actually touched.

Two things are common in the people I've talked to about sexual abuse. One: the belief they were to blame for it somehow, and thus were 'bad to the bone' even as tiny humans. Two: many people I've spoken with *did tell* a Responsible Adult. And they either weren't believed ('you're so imaginative!' or 'you're such a drama queen'), or they were accused of actually encouraging it.

This seems common particularly when a family member was involved in the abuse (which they weren't, in any of my experiences). When the molestation involves a relative, the urge to bury it, rather than bring it to light, is scarily common.

And so the child is given the rock to hold forevermore, because the Responsible Adult won't share the weight of it. It's very easy to say to a child: 'it was just a dream' or 'you're exaggerating', and sweep it under the family-preserving rug.

As if a nine-year-old would ever exaggerate about a 50-year-old getting into their bed and pressing up against them. Or fantasise about it, for that matter, and then confuse the fantasia with reality.

It's often the *not being believed* – the *you imagined it* or the *you brought it upon yourself* subtext – that tears a tiny hole in a tiny soul, more so than the act itself. Because when you try to give a trusted adult that rock, and they refuse it, or even turn it into a weapon against you, you become a miniature human who feels utterly unprotected.

If you relate to this, I'm sorry. I can't take that rock from you, but please allow me to hold it with you for a while. I believe you. And *of course* you played no part in it whatsoever. No child should ever feel responsible for a grown adult's actions.

Self-parenting

Finally, many ACE-survivors have what therapists call a 'critical parent' voice in their heads. Often, this is an echo of an actual parent, but sometimes it's a blend of both, or a teacher, or a grandparent, or any significant figure. It's that snarky voice that trash-talks us every time we do something 'wrong'. That says we're lazy, stupid, selfish good-for-nothing gobshites.

Often we think we need the subtle snarl of the 'critical parent' to get shit done, or stay on the right road, or be good people. In particular, I was attached to my 'you're lazy' narrative, given I thought it put a rocket up my ass. I thought that, without it, I'd never get anything done ever again.

So, I was astonished to discover that when I replaced this with a 'nurturing parent' vibe of, 'c'mon pumpkin, up you get, you can do this!', I actually got *more done*. But of course I did. I don't know why I was surprised. Positive reinforcement is more effective, we know that now. It's in all of the most recent parenting books. And parenting yourself is no exception.

When we crave a drink, that 'critical parent' tends to blast us like a bull horn with 'don't be so stupid!' or 'have you learned nothing?!' But it may be more helpful to talk to the part of us that wants a drink as if it's a small child determined to go to the supermarket in midwinter wearing a unicorn swimsuit and sparkly shoes. 'Not a good idea, sweetie' or 'That's not for the best'. Kind and nurturing, rather than impatient and scowling.

With my 'nurturing parent' robes on, I went back to that room, to my 12-year-old self, who thinks everyone hates her, who feels unloveable, and I gave her the biggest hug. I told her she's worthy of love, even when she's a twonk. I tell her everything's going to be OK. Well, it won't be for a long while. She will seek comfort in bottles and the feeling of 'I am enough' between the sheets. *But eventually, it will be OK poppet, it really will.*

Ironically, one of my acts as a self-parent was to quit therapy. I did it weekly, for six months. After each session, I had a therapy hangover. For 24 hours, I felt wan, blue, sometimes even on the brink of despair. Then I would buoy back up and feel lighter. But my 'therapy hangover' didn't mean it wasn't working. It meant it *was.* I was unpacking all of my rocks and showing someone for the first time, which was tiring and testing.

But then I left. I didn't want to stay in the inky depths of childhood trauma therapy forevermore. A self-parent knows when to stop, when enough is enough, and when to come back up to the sunnier waters. I couldn't live down there indefinitely; it was too intense. I'll go back to therapy for any other personal challenges, but my childhood has now been laid to rest. Your self-parent will know what's right for you, once you tap into them.

We can't 'fix' a trauma-punctuated childhood. There's no 'undo' button. We've been there and got the T-shirt, kiddos. But we can change our future. Because we're not little any more. We're big now.

Funny thing, dear reader. Knowing our way intimately around our ACEs, our wiring, our network, our buttons, may just make us better able to fully love. Not just ourselves, but others too.

'It was as though he could not unlock his love until he had unlocked his grief'

Philippa Perry,
The Book You Wish Your Parents Had Read

NOTES ON SOBER FLIRTING

Bars and nightclubs are living, breathing Tinders/Grindrs that we no longer access into the portions of the night when everyone gets a bit handsy. Back then, we didn't need to swipe right. We just looked right.

We didn't need to exchange 310 messages and have a nutter-check phone call before finally meeting; we just met. Digital fireworks to denote a match? Nah. The nearness of them triggers bodily fireworks, if only in your undercrackers.

When you're sober and spend approximate 20 hours *less* a week in the twilit bedlam of bars, and virtually no time in the 3D Fumble of nightclubs, it is undeniably harder to meet, to flirt, to pick up. (Don't even get us started on life post-Covid.)

I met dozens of new potential suitors a week when I was drinking. Many of whom were saved on my phone under interesting names like 'Red Lion chap' or 'Weird train guy'. I recently did a search in my messages and a message chain from 'Molecule Dude' showed up. Oh crap. *Here we go*, I thought.

I opened it as one might handle a grenade, expecting him to be a Ghost of Clublands Past. Nope. Somebody I bought an art print off, arranging delivery. How unbelievably wholesome, rather than wanton.

But if you allow yourself to flirt in a different way, to 'flip it', like a razorfish (unconstrained by horizontal fish laws, these bad boys can swim vertically too), you'll find there are plenty of fish also doing it this way. Picking up people in the bakery line. Or at our co-working space. Or in the park.

As sobers, we learn how to flirt sunshine warm sober. Which actually negates much of the need for apps, the braver you get.

The older I get, the more I realise (having had approximately 156 internet dates) that apps are often introducing us to people we ought not to meet.

If they live on the street over and your social lives have never overlapped, like Venn diagrams, then perhaps *they weren't supposed to*. Perhaps you two like different sorts of people and different sorts of things. They're more of a 'smoke weed outside a gig' type, while you're more of a spinning-and-brunch character. It's my firm belief that people who meet organically and outside alcohol-centric environments, whether through friends-of-friends, in a climbing centre or at a gallery opening, tend to be more compatible.

Why? It's not last-orders panic shopping. 'Quick, the lights have gone up, grab the nearest warm body!', whom you chose purely based on BMI and cheekbones, rather than the attributes that last: wit and grit. And nor is it 'high investment', in that you've already spent four hours messaging this Godforsaken person, so you try to fancy them, even though you probably wouldn't otherwise.

Ultimately, friends, even though teetotalling means less suitors, the sober matches you do get are superior. Because the chemistry is not co-created by ethanol. And the party in our pants is not sponsored by sauvignon blanc.

KIDS: UNDERAGE DRINKING MEANS HIGHER ADDICTION

Aged 14, I spend the night on a roundabout in Wolverhampton.

Tonight, I am going to The Dorchester nightclub with my friend, Cerys. The Dorch, for short, is a mezzanined den of underage iniquity. All we have to do to get in is robotically recite a date of birth – twice – that makes us slightly over 18 (bang on 18 is a no-no; every tearaway knows that, 19 is the sweet spot), and flash an ill-gotten student railcard/ forged university library card.

Even though we are more underage than most, with our bee-sting tits and non-existent hips, Cerys and I never have a problem getting in. The doorman reportedly fancies me, which greases the wheels. (In fact, I'd started going to The Dorch when I was 13. When I turn 16, the doorman will make it clear he expects payment, so I give him a hand job in his souped-up boy racer in the car park. The romance!)

To ready ourselves, 14-year old Cerys and I put on our flowery dresses, our Rimmel Heather Shimmer lipstick, douse ourselves with White Musk body spray and push our silver nose studs in, jangling two 45p bus fares out of my fat silver piggy bank.

We've told my mother we're watching a film and we tiptoe as ballet-like as you can in cherry-red Doc Martens across the flat roof outside my bedroom window, drop down into the local park, stifling giggles, and clomp our way through a pitch-black park (safety first!) to the number 1 bus.

A litre of White Lightning later, we have the requisite swagger of the lost fifth and sixth members of Sleeper. We spend the night head-nodding to The Stone Roses, jumping around to House of Pain, yelling along to *The Levellers* about there being no other way, and coercing wannabe Evan Dandos into buying us drinks.

But then, we miss the last bus home. And a £20 taxi home to Dudley is about as achievable on our budget as a private jet. Standing there, at the barren bus stop, we're forced to contemplate our fate of a five-hour wait until the morning buses resume.

We stand in a phone box for a while, debating who we can legitimately rouse – without major consequence – at 2am. Ummm. No one. We can't call either of our parents as we'll bring nuclear war upon our 14-year-old heads. All of our friends will be in bed. Besides, mobile phones are still the reserve of rappers or CEOs with BMWs, so we don't have a direct line to them.

Thankfully, it's been the kind of balmy British day that entices everyone to get their kit off and toast their tits. The fried air outside Chicken Licken holds the heat, and the pavement is warm to the touch. But, there's a catch. Wolverhampton post-midnight is about as safe as Wormwood Scrubs. We won't be cold, but we could be killed.

The adventure. I'm electrified by it.

'I know!' I exclaim. I point at a straggly-bush-covered roundabout. 'Let's hide in there.' (As plans go, I still think it was equal parts idiocy and ingenuity. Think about it. How many serial killers, or paedophiles, or berserk Samurai-sword-wielders, are likely to take a shortcut through a roundabout, in case there might be teenage prey there? Zilch.)

So, we buy a loaf of white bread from the 24-hour petrol station with our remaining 50p and hunker down for the night in our roundabout bed. Immersed in a road-traffic and hedge-filtered headlight ASMR lullaby, we tear off chunks of bread and lob them into each other's gobs as if we're oversized ducks.

***

That night was probably the most fun I've ever had camping. (The attraction of camping mystifies me.) And yet we were kids. Actual kids. When I look at 14-year-olds now, all knees, elbows and gobby hormones play-fighting with the linger of soft childishness, I feel confronted by what I was doing at their exact age. The thought of what could have happened to us that night makes my spine contract, my blood freeze.

A landmark 1998 US study found that those who start drinking at age 15 or younger are *four times* more likely to become addicted than those who start drinking at 21. (But who starts drinking at 21?! Some people actually do. I *know*.)

Regardless of how unrealistic 21 is, 18 as a drinking start might not be too moonshot, right? And the fact is, the rates of addiction likelihood 'reduce by 4% and 5% with each year drug use onset was delayed', the study said. So a teen who starts drinking at 18 rather than 14 is up to 20 per cent *less likely* to go on to become addicted. I'll take those odds.

'The data is crystal clear on the incidence between early pick-up and higher rates of addiction later,' says Dr Judith Grisel. Why, I ask? 'Younger people are better at learning anything, and that includes addiction.'

'Yes, the brain "learns" addiction, even though we associate learning with positivity,' Dr Grisel says. 'The earlier we start anything, the more we take to it, whether it's learning a language, playing an instrument, or playing a sport.'

'The earlier the child picks up the substance, the more plastic and malleable their brains are,' she says, 'and the more likely they are to learn to use it in an addictive manner. Our brains have more neuroplasticity at 15 than 18.'

The reason for pick-up is often those Godforsaken ACEs again. Remember how, earlier, Dr Grisel said that ACEs and early use are proxies? And therefore almost indistinguishable? Yup, that.

'The trauma is often the catalyst for teen pick-up,' she says. 'Which then leads to the later dependence. So, it would be more accurate, in my opinion, to say that the early use is the strongest predictor. Even though the data leads us to the ACEs.' In-ter-est-ing.

In training to be drinkers

My underage drinking stories may make me sound feral, but I was actually pretty sedate next to some of the people I hung out with. All of whom were birthed into a privileged cabbage patch. Regardless of our middle-class, scented-candle home lives, we were all delinquents. Our drinking careers were in full, smells-like-teen-spirit swing by the time we were 13.

By 14, we were all nightclubbing on the regular. All of us dated small-time dealers at some point. That's just what we were doing. We were also wearing Smashing Pumpkins T-shirts and Vans, reading John Donne and Jane Austen, and working our asses off on getting not just As but A*s. Was that just what teens in the Nineties did? I don't know.

I've witnessed kids who are *under ten* being given sips of beer out of Daddy's glass, or a finger of fizz at Xmas, or a suck on a parental finger dipped in Irish cream. We train our kids to grow up to be drinkers. We assume they'll drink. And I've even witnessed teens-of-age who choose not to drink getting a hard time from their parents (in Ireland, which is famously boozy). 'Lighten up, wouldja?! Have a beer!'

Of course, as with almost everything, I've been guilty of this underage drink-training myself. When I was 27, I attended a family party in a chocolate-box Irish cottage, which involved drinking, tall tales, an open fire and poker. My distant cousin's 15-year-old daughter was there, along with her friend. They were quizzing me about the magazine industry, eyes wide at the stories I was telling of photo shoots, freebies and demands from A-list publicists.

'I'm getting a drink, do you want one?' I said, after a half hour of chat. 'Oh, we'll just have lemonade, we're only 15,' one responded. 'I can sneak some cider into that if you like?' I responded, nudge-wink conspiratorial, playing the cool older chick. I went on to feed them at least three lemonade-ciders each, while telling them how great drinking was.

Then one puked outside. Her father interrogated both of them as to what they'd drunk, and how. I saw his furious gaze land on me from across the room. *Uh oh. Busted.* He pulled me outside into the winter chill, to give me a dressing down I'll never forget.

There I stood, in the romantically frost-laced garden, jutting my bottom lip like a disgruntled child, while he fired phrases like 'irresponsible adult' and 'bad example' into the freezing air, while the words hung there in accusatory clouds. I stared at the clouds, rather than his furious face.

The irony was, both of us were steaming that night in the garden, not just me. Sneaking drinks to teens is irrefutably wrong, but by getting legless on a regular basis, many of us are unwittingly colluding in the not-so-subliminal messaging of 'this is what adults do to have fun'. I think about that often; how many times I have been a rat-arsed anti-hero for the youngsters in my huge Irish family. Too many times to count.

Teentotallers

But the future looks bright. Different. 'Teentotallers' is now a buzz phrase. Indeed, 'Twentytotalling' is also a thing, if less catchy. In 2018, a survey of 10,000 18-to-24-year-olds turned up something startling to the press, triggering an avalanche of headlines. Nearly a third of them – 29 per cent – don't drink (up from 18 per cent in 2005).

A study by the National Union of Students found that not only do a lot of young people not drink, they've *never* drunk. A fifth of undergraduates have never drunk alcohol, the survey found. But this doesn't change the fact that 70 per cent of them felt pressured to drink.

Seventy per cent is alarming, but still an improvement. When I was at university, I'm guessing this would have been 99 per cent. Our leisure time was exclusively spent out ('out-out' wasn't a thing yet. Frankly, every night was out-out) at 'Frenzy', 'Beer pong', 'VodBull' or 'Fever'. Which all pretty much sound like maladies that would have you sent to an asylum in the early 1900s for a spot of straitjackets 'n' leeches.

If I'd yelled, 'No ta, I'm not drinking' at a mate during one of those 99p-a-pint nights, I'm fairly sure my fellow students would have 'Dentist Chaired' me with a bottle of hard cider. And make no mistake: I would have done the same to them.

I wanted to know more about this. So I talked to the early sober adopters: Generation Z, those aged 18 to 24. I asked: why are a third of you teetotal? And is the struggle real, or is peer pressure improving?

Most prominently, I was told that Gen Z-ers have to work hard to find sober friends, just like the rest of us. 'These stats don't feel representative of my experience!' 21-year-old Ella told me. 'I wonder if perhaps there's a relationship between non-drinking and engaging in surveys or research?!'

She gets pushback on quitting so young. 'The most common reaction I get to my non-drinking is: "you have your whole life ahead of you; you'll be missing out". The irony is that, if I don't remember these experiences, I miss out!' she laughs.

However, there are positives. 'My fifty-something parents have never been binge drinkers, like me, so they can't understand why I'm sober. However, my previous housemates (twenties/early thirties) were much more understanding. Online sober communities have been an incredible tool for meeting people – especially Sober & Social and Sober Girl Society.'

Many teentotallers grew up watching their parents drink and thought 'no ta'. This was 23-year-old Rob's experience. 'Both my dad's Guinness and mum's wine smelt dreadful to me. By 16 I hadn't heard good things about it, so I just decided to carry on. I'm now in my early twenties and don't plan on ever trying it. Explaining it to others is weird as I don't have a 'proper' reason (not that I need one) other than I'm just not interested in it at all.'

Like Ella, 18-year-old Becky has found that her peers tend to be pretty understanding. 'During my first Christmas sober, I still went out to the theatre, hung out with my mates and went out on Christmas Eve. I felt so empowered. At first, I felt so nervous. But once I explained why I wasn't drinking (anxiety, not being in control, the regret and shame) my friends completely understood. Most of them actually felt the same way.'

Meanwhile, 19-year-old Leona's been given some grief, but says the positives are worth it. 'I'm a year sober after ending up in situations that were at best embarrassing and, at worst, plain dangerous,' she reveals. 'It can be a challenge to make new friends at uni. Some of my peers laugh, ask why I don't drink, then tell me I should. It can be a little lonely when everyone else is planning to drink, and all you want to do is have a natter and admire teapots on a café crawl. It's improved my mental health tenfold, though, and I have some wonderfully supportive people on my side.'

Teddy bear's champagne breakfast

Good news for all of my Gen Z case studies and readers: there's a flipside to the neuroplasticity associated with early pick-up, says Dr Grisel. 'The risk of addiction *is* higher the younger you pick up, yes, but it's also easier to recover quickly if you quit drinking in your early twenties.'

'The brain's development slows down at 21, but the brain doesn't really mature until 25,' she adds. Given the brain is still more 'plastic' and changeable before 25, Dr Grisel says that those who quit young tend to have a slightly easier time with it. So those *absolute heroes* who quit young have the right idea.

To finish, I'll say this. Do me a favour the next time you see someone 'mock drinking' with their nine-year-old on Facebook. When they post a picture of them and their kid in front of a champagne breakfast, replete with vintage glassware, with teddy bears as guests. Don't like it. Don't press heart. Don't comment: 'cute!' Equally, don't tell them to take it down either, because that will just piss them off.

However, if you know them well, do perhaps tell them in a roundabout 'oh isn't this interesting' manner about underage drinking and how it predicts higher addiction. It might spark a realisation. We need much more awareness around this. Not *judgement*: awareness.

'What's the harm?!' people cry. 'The liquid in their champagne flute is water!' But when we engage in this pretend-play, this mock-drinking, this faux-cheersing with kids, this is what we're saying: 'One day, my peach, one day you shall have champagne too. And won't you be lucky, when that day comes!' We're setting up the "alcohol: reward" association incredibly early. We're accelerating their drinking.

Alcohol is a loaded gun for untimely deaths in the young. A 2016 World Health Organization study found that alcohol was responsible for one in four deaths among 16–24-year-olds.

'There is a particular danger point for dying the night you become a legal drinker – 18 in the UK, 21 in the US – because people press drinks on the young person, thinking they are being nice,' says Professor David Nutt. 'Of course, children will do what you do, not what you say... Don't be the person who buys them drink.'

Why on earth are we encouraging our kids to grow up to be drinkers – and even giving them drinks when they're underage – in light of all this? How's about teaching them how *not to* drink during social events, given they'll be getting enough pressure from elsewhere *to drink*?

In a truly bizarre twist, a reader, Eleanor, told this story. She and her husband no longer drink, so they don't keep alcohol in the house. 'People often ask if I'm worried my children will grow up to be addicted to alcohol because they won't have been exposed to it?'

This twisty-turny logic (*not logic*) says that exposure inoculates against addiction, when it's quite the opposite. A house heaving with booze makes early pick-up intensely *more likely*. Kids can't buy alcohol, and strangers are unlikely to buy it for them (these days; not so in the Nineties), so if it's not in the home within reach, surely it means they're more likely to wait until they're of legal drinking age-ish (if they drink at all). Logically, Eleanor and her husband are actually lowering their kids' chances of becoming addicted.

'These people say "but you're not normalising alcohol!"' Eleanor adds. 'But I don't want to normalise alcohol. When I talk to my kids about alcohol, I talk about it like any other drug. About what it does to your brain; that it's addictive. I don't wag my finger and say "never drink", but I'm not going to teach them that alcohol is a necessary rite of passage either.'

WHY ARE PREGNANT WOMEN STILL TOLD 'ONE WON'T HURT'?

I'm not surprised that 4 in 10 Brits drink during pregnancy. I would've, had I fallen pregnant when I was still drinking. And what's more, I would have been encouraged to, by the lion's share of society.

I was at a baby shower recently and witnessed the chorus of 'one won't hurt!' toward the mother-to-be, who eventually gave in and reluctantly sipped a glass of sauvignon blanc. She didn't finish it. I strongly suspect she didn't want it in the first place.

Up until a few years ago, the received wisdom was indeed that one or two drinks a week was fine. But the new NHS advice, based on up-to-date evidence, is that the 'safest approach is not to drink at all, to keep risks to your baby to a minimum'.

In 2017, the British Medical Journal said that a meta-analysis of 26 studies showed that 'drinking up to four units a week while pregnant, on average, was associated with an 8 per cent higher risk of having a small baby, compared with drinking no alcohol at all. There was also some evidence of a heightened risk of premature birth, but this was less clear.'

Hence the 'none is best' advice. Yet the 'one won't hurt!' drink-pushing persists. I wonder if it's time for some sort of public health campaign in order to make the NHS advice crystal clear – to not just pregnant women, but also those around them.

Conflicting messages given to the pregnant

In autumn 2017, there was a glut of newspaper headlines that appeared to contradict the new 'don't drink when pregnant' NHS guidelines as hysterical. Even the right-on, usually careful *Guardian* ran with the headline 'Little evidence that light drinking in pregnancy is harmful, say experts'.

It turns out that the new study, from the University of Bristol, was flagging an 'absence of evidence' not an 'evidence of absence'. It was a call for more research. 'Our extensive review shows that this specific question is not being researched thoroughly enough, if at all,' the study's leaders wrote in the *BMJ*.

It was entirely misrepresented by the press. Manipulated into clickbait. If a pregnant woman had simply scanned the headline and the first few paragraphs, thcy would have concluded that there's little evidence that light drinking can harm their baby.

A responsible headline would have been 'Experts call for research into whether light drinking is harmful while pregnant'. That would have summed up what the study was *actually* saying. But maybe it would have garnered less clicks.

The press ought to be reporting things responsibly, rather than angling for traffic over factual accuracy. And, as a society, we should be helping pregnant women not to drink, rather than peer-pressuring them into it.

I'm not a parent, nor have I ever been pregnant, so I asked some pregnant women and mothers to tell me: what were your experiences like drinking/not drinking while pregnant? What advice were you given and what pressures did you feel?

'I felt like my non-drinking made other mothers feel judged'

HOLLY SAYS:

'I was six months pregnant during my third pregnancy, and out for lunch with ex-workmates. I ordered a soft drink. "Oh, you're not going to have a drink? Bella did," one said. She gestured to Bella, who'd had two mimosas at every work lunch we'd had during pregnancy. I said no thanks. And then she said, "But doctors say it's fine."

I ended up making other excuses for my non-drinking like, "I've got a headache" or "I'm really tired" because it didn't seem to be a good enough excuse to say "I'm growing a tiny person."

I never pushed back on those who pushed booze because I didn't want other women to feel judged that they *had* drank while pregnant. I actually enjoyed not drinking while pregnant – it took the internal battle of whether to drink or not totally off the table.

When I was breastfeeding, the pressure continued. One friend told me that I couldn't eat onions while breastfeeding my six-week-old, but she was also pushing champagne on me. "If you're nursing it's OK, because by the time the alcohol is in your system it's OK." I'd just have a few sips to avoid the conflict and keep everyone quiet.

I've been sober for two years now and I still haven't told my friends I no longer drink. I'm scared. And yet not drinking has helped me a million per cent. While drinking I was snappy and spent my weekends miserable, yelling at the kids to hurry up and get into bed so that I could have a drink. Now, I'm much calmer.'

'A midwife recommended drinking during labour'

CAROLINE SAYS:

'I'm a first time mum-to-be and quit drinking 18 months before falling pregnant. It's surprised me how much drinking has come up among pregnant women. I read a book that had a whole section on how to pretend you're drinking during the first trimester.

Lots of sources recommend packing a bottle of champagne in the hospital bag. I heard a midwife on a podcast recommend drinking a couple of glasses of wine during labour to relax – her logic was that given Pethidine is an opiate, it can't be any worse than that.

Four out of five meet-ups with my antenatal group have discussed drinking – how much they miss it, how much they are looking forward to doing so again. "I miss lying on my stomach," I said. Another chipped in with: "I just miss wine so much," and there was such longing in her face. I have lots of compassion for that, as that would have been me, before I quit.

I haven't been asked whether I miss drinking while pregnant, so I'd have to volunteer it and say "I actually don't drink", so I haven't said anything. I don't want them to feel judged. If someone curious starts the conversation, I'm here.

The very first thing our breastfeeding counsellor said was, "Yes, you can drink alcohol." But what's the logic? If everything you eat or drink comes through the breast milk, like caffeine, how come booze doesn't?

I'm looking forward to being an alcohol-free mother. Author Annie Grace said that she raised two babies while drinking and found the sleepless nights horrific. But her recent daughter was raised while she was alcohol-free – and she said the sleepless nights were actually manageable. That's a relief!'

'I'm haunted by the time I had two glasses while pregnant'

KATIE SAYS:

'Eight months after my son Seb arrived earthside, we noticed some unusual mannerisms. His arms were always up – bent at the elbow and flexed. Doctors called it the "I win" position. We just thought it was cute. But a month or two later, he'd be sitting in his high chair and still doing it. He would grab his food, then his arms would go right back up.

I went to have him checked out by a paediatrician. One of her questions was, "Did you drink during pregnancy?" I lied and said no. She said that the arm movement and the scissoring of his legs were markers for cerebral palsy.

I was barely taking it all in because I kept thinking, "I've done this. This was the alcohol." It was very confronting. Seb was my second baby so I was more blasé during pregnancy. I had lots of people around me saying "one won't hurt". And that "one glass of wine when you're pregnant is like giving your baby one drop of wine in a swimming pool".

I knew it was rubbish, but I wanted the glass of champagne, so I listened to the person who said it was fine to have it. Once in particular I had two glasses, but they were big glasses. And this "two glasses" moment was now replaying over and over in my mind, on an awful loop.

We took Seb to see a professor at a children's hospital for a second opinion. Again, he asked, "Did you drink during pregnancy?" It wasn't a 50-question survey; it was one of only six questions. Again, I lied and said no. I decided telling the truth wasn't going to change anything about Seb's condition.

The second doctor arrived at the same conclusion: cerebral

palsy. Luckily, we received early intervention and after a year of intensive daily physio, Seb is fine.

The guilt I felt during that year is something I have never gotten over. It was a constant, sick dread. And I actually drank more, because of it. But then I finally realised, "why am I putting this stuff in my body, given it potentially caused my child's disability?"

I'll never know if it *was* the alcohol or not, that caused Seb's cerebral palsy. Nonetheless, whenever I hear people saying "one won't hurt" to a pregnant woman, I cringe and want to shout my story from the rooftops. A glass is not worth the guilt and "what ifs" afterward. Nine months is such a short time in the grand scheme.'

***

STONE COLD VS SUNSHINE WARM SUMMER

STONE COLD DRUNK SUMMER

JUNE 2004

There's a knock at the door. Ugh. I roll out of bed, pull a dressing gown on (why is it wet? And why is it so big?) and go to answer it.

The hotel maid, insultingly pin-neat and shiny. 'Good morning, Madam! Your clothes, Madam. From room 125.'

My mouth drops open as she hands me a plastic bag. Inside are the clothes I was wearing last night, but they're full of sea and sand. I try to say something, but all that comes out is a squeak.

'Have a nice...' starts the maid, but I shut the door in her face. I am so ablaze with shame, I can't let her finish the nicety. My heart has dropped like a free-falling elevator.

I sit on the edge of the bed, the bag of clothes in my lap, and touch my hair. It's loaded with salt. I think, hard.

OK, so my holiday companion and I drank several cocktails. Roger that. Then I made a beeline for a mostly male French running team, also staying at our hotel, who I'd seen doing sand-running drills on the beach. 'Snap me off a piece of that', I'd thought, watching them. So next thing, I was sitting with the running team, drinking, minus my plus one. Gotcha.

What happened then? All I have are flashes, as if a dark room is illuminated briefly by a flash camera. Flash – 'I have never' drinking game. Flash – howls of laughter. Flash – playing poker back in their room. Flash – me trying to get them to play for money. Flash – getting closer to one of them, Erik. Flash – feeling Erik's hard runner's thigh against mine.

*And then. Flash, flash, flash – this particular memory sequence is
stronger. At approximately 2am, myself and five of the men decided
it was a super idea to strip down to our pants and race into the Indian
Ocean, watched by a bemused hotel guard, who said something into a
walkie-talkie and then decided to let our infantile Western spectacle
play out.*

*We swam out to a tarpaulin-covered yacht, hauled our soaking
bodies onto the deck and stared at the pinhead-star canopy above. This.
This was a story, I told myself, as Erik felt for my hand.*

*As we swam back, giggling like children, I felt it. The thing I want
from this and every night out. The belonging. The togetherness. I belong
to this running team, and they to me, now that we've shared this illicit
2am swim. I never want this spell to be broken. I know morning will
break it. The night is the only place it exists.*

*After this, I only have one more flash. Flash – myself and Erik in
the shower, naked, kissing. That's it. That's all I have. I can only assume
that this is his hotel gown that drowns me, and that I left his room
without my clothes.*

*I spend the rest of the day imagining that the hotel staff are
whispering about me, trading stories about my 2am swim and my wet,
sandy clothes, ('what a slut'), when the reality is, they probably don't
give a toss. They have work to do. The antics of a spoilt British bird are
the least of their concerns.*

*I think and think, but no more comes back. I still only have around
eight jigsaw puzzle pieces from last night, when there ought to be 30.*

*That evening, I handwash the heavy sand out of my clothes. And I
find a note, now wet, at the bottom. It's from Erik.*

'Last night was unforgettable.'

SUNSHINE WARM SOBER SUMMER

JULY 2020

Group meetings outside have finally been endorsed by the British government. I never thought I'd write that sentence. It feels so Orwellian, but these are the strangelands in which we now live. (I often wonder what we would make of Summer 2020 Britain if we were airlifted into it from NYE 2019.)

I have been invited to a BBQ on the beach by a man I like. I'm nervous. I put one foot in front of the other and chant 'just get there, just get there, just get there', as I know now that the before bit is always the most challenging. Once I'm there, I'm pretty much golden.

I bond with a new female friend, Heather. We eat veggie burgers. Somebody manages to sprain an ankle falling off a paddleboard. He will become a friend too. We laugh, a lot. We discuss tattoos. Myself and the man I like exchange shy, lingering looks.

And then, something happens. The sun shaft-streams through the clouds, the BBQ smokes roasted pepper and a retro 'Driving songs for Dad' song drops. 'The Boys of Summer' by Don Henley. Tune! We turn it up.

Everyone falls silent for the melodramatic Eighties guitar music solo. There's definitely a perm playing this guitar. People close their eyes. Sway. And as the vocals start, three of us sing along, fingers in the air. 'Nobody on the road, nobody on the beach/I feel it in the air, the summer's out of reach.' Somebody gets up and does a twirl.

It's here! The moment. The togetherness. The clan-style belonging. That for two decades I thought was impossible without alcohol.

Later, I say goodbye to the man I like. The others, sensing that there is something hatching, give us some privacy. We text the next day. We start dating the week after. It will be another six weeks before he sees me naked. And two months before we sleep together.

Best of all, I'll remember every single thing.

BURNING QUESTION: IS ADDICTION GENETIC?

Dr Julia Lewis: 'There are certain genes that increase your risk of addiction, yes; some of which are related to the metabolism of alcohol or things like the signalling pathways in the brain that alcohol affects. But it's not black and white. The classic adoption study is usually cited, where the sons of fathers *with* an alcohol dependence were raised away from their fathers, in families *without* an alcohol dependence issue. Still, they were generally found to be two to three times more likely to develop an addiction than those without the genes of an alcohol-dependent parent. Nonetheless, this wasn't *always* the case. Genes are not a foregone conclusion; they can just sometimes tip the scales.'

Dr David Nutt says: 'Some elements of it are. Some genetically inherited characteristics make you vulnerable, such as impulsivity, anxiety or reward sensitivity. There's quite a strong concordance in identical twins that backs this up.'

Dr Marc Lewis says: 'No, but there are personality characteristics that are partly hereditary that can predispose towards addiction. For instance, anxiety and introversion can predispose towards addiction, but also the opposite personality traits can predispose as well; such as risk-taking and impulsive behaviour.'

Dr Judith Grisel says: 'There's much we still don't know, but we do know that around half the risk comes from genetic factors. Anxiety disorders, for instance, which are partly hereditary. The easily bored are more prone to marijuana use, while the anxious find that alcohol works for their anxiety problem. Until it starts to exacerbate it. Sensitivity to alcohol is genetic too. Those people who are a 'lightweight' or 'cheap date'? They're unable to metabolise alcohol as efficiently, which means their bodies are effectively protecting them from addiction. This comes down to a particular protein in a receptor. So, being able to drink a lot – or less severe hangovers – may seem like a good thing, but they're actually a predictor for later addiction.'

IS IT HARDER FOR MEN TO GET SOBER?

Of late, it's become a twisted badge for feminist rebellion to swill a whiskey sour, but for decades – centuries, even – before that, it was a badge for masculinity to be a big drinker.

Beyond 'toxic masculinity', there's also 'intoxicated masculinity' – given all of the dunderheadedness around inhaling a yard of ale and being 'macho', or downing pints and putting them on top of your head, like an absurd glass hat. Even ordering a half a lager in a pub can summon rambunctious jibes of 'pussy' or 'sissy', let alone ordering *no lager at all*. Getting sober is hard enough without your positive lifestyle choice being treated as an insult to your gender. It's just binary bullshit.

I think this 'beer pressure' often makes it harder for men to get sober. So, I asked some of them about it.

'As a younger man, getting drunk was almost a sport in itself. Friendships are built around it. All the stories we share as men involved drunken antics, sex, or both. The habit, the culture, endures.'

Daniel

'It was a big help for me when alcohol-free beer became more prevalent in pubs, restaurants and even the football stadium. Once I had an alcohol-free beer in my hand, the comments reduced significantly and then pretty much completely. I would go so far as to say that, without alcohol-free beer, I probably would have failed going sober. I removed a few toxic friends and now everyone in my circle is supportive.'

Caleb

'Because of perceptions of masculinity, being sober can make you feel weak in a peer group. It feels hard in the workplace, especially for me in the Army, where so much of our identity and gravitas can be wrapped up in our social and outwardly visible 'selves'. Overcoming all that doubt and anxiety to change your identity is like jumping into an ice pool of cold shock. But it's been worth it. The most surprising thing is just how much people want to help once you reach out. Nine times out of ten, other men are like, "Fair play", because deep down, they know the challenge involved.'

Thomas

'I always associated hard drinking with creativity rather than laddish culture *per se*. I drank because the majority of my creative heroes did so. Hemingway and Kerouac in particular. It was a wonderland rabbit hole where I would descend daily to be king, genius, savant. I hid there for decades. Only now, realising that my days on earth are increasingly scarce, have I found the courage to think for myself. The hardest part by far, though, is my partner mourning our joint evenings in wine bars sharing a bottle of red. That separation of experience required far more courage.'

Ben

'As a straight man who loves sports, nearly everything I enjoy doing is surrounded by booze. Golfing, sports bars, watching a game, softball, etc. The more guys around, the stronger the pressure becomes. The group will essentially bond over making fun of the non-drinker and telling their war stories about drinking. I've found that abstaining altogether is easier (and more enjoyable) than leaving the door open a little.'

Eric

ACTUAL CRAVINGS VS DIFFICULT EMOTIONS

One of the most common questions I get is, 'Do you still crave it'? And the answer is: no, I bloody well don't. I crave it like a crocodile-attack survivor craves a candlelit dinner with a crocodile. Nonetheless, what I do still have is *that* urge. That twitch. That scratch. That universally experienced urgency to flee my own skin by reaching for a quick fix. A fast lane, an easy button, an 'uncomfortable feelings' escape chute.

Others who are long-term sober may well interpret those emotions as cravings. Particularly if they subscribe to the notion that any discomfort is a craving. Whatever floats your boat, Toto. Conflicting opinions and interpretations are our birthright.

Personally, though, I know this: when I don't see every uncomfortable emotion as a craving, I feel much safer from alcohol. I am still vigilant for cravings, but I know the difference between emotions and cravings. And to name these emotions for what they are: anxiety, anger, frustration, despair, insecurity, jealousy, fear. I used alcohol to medicate these emotions for 21 years, but it doesn't mean the emotion *is* the craving.

These emotions are universal, central to the human condition. They have been since the dawn of us. Ever since we were scratching pictures of fire and buffalo into cave walls, we've tried to dodge them. People will always try to drink, smoke, toke, shag, gamble, shop, eat, not eat and work their way out of feeling what they're feeling.

But then, sometimes the feeling is a craving for alcohol. I got them many, many times in the first few years. You'll know a craving because it's 2D, childish and about as rational and subtle as a cartoon walloping you over the head with a mallet. 'Gimme!' cravings cry. 'Want now!' They're the irrational wrestling the rational in a headlock. They're Homer vs Lisa Simpson, Cookie Monster vs Big Bird, Scrappy Doo vs Daphne. They're your short-term self throwing down with your long-term self. And the secret, of course, is to have your long-term self win in that tug o' war. But then you know that, if you're already successfully sober.

A dear friend of mine's motto was, 'What would morning Eve think about that?' By asking that very simple-yet-powerful question, she gave her long-term self more power. She brought her prefrontal cortex online, rather than letting her primal, emotion-driven amygdala call the shots. Her inner Lisa just overruled her inner Homer (age doesn't necessarily denote wisdom). Genius.

There was a brilliant *Humans of New York* recently where the interviewed Human said that given a life do-over she'd party less, because 'there are two selves. There's your short-term self, and there's your long-term self. And if you're only true to your short-term self, your long-term self slowly decays.'

And when it's an uncomfortable emotion?

In early recovery, it *was* the right thing for me to reach out, text someone, see someone, or tap into a group (whether online or IRL) every time I experienced an emotion that felt like a craving. But now? I sit through them. Unless there's something fierce moving through me, I tend to manage my emotions myself.

Of course, I had help learning how to do this in the first place. Mindfulness taught me the power of naming emotions to disarm them. And then my therapist taught me to locate the size, shape and whereabouts of discomfort in the body. My fear of abandonment, for instance, feels like a grey stone in the pit of my stomach. My anxiety feels smoky, like heartburn and nausea rising.

Most of my uncomfortable emotions manifest in my gut. For so very long 'butterflies in the stomach' or a 'gut instinct' were assumed to be metaphorical. An airy-fairy way of describing that which lived in the brain. But we now know that emotions live in the gut *and* the brain. Emotions in the amygdala trigger gut problems, and vice versa.

I don't seek external comfort, on the whole, nowadays. I can have a blue day – even a blue few days– without telling anyone. I don't *need* to any more. My emotions, my moods, are my responsibility. What's more, it's not much fun for our friends or family to mostly hear from us when we're clobbered by a negative emotion.

I recently went through a spell of red-hot romantic jealousy, which blazed through my brain like a forest fire, and was outrageously irrational. 'I think it's one of the flipsides of having an overactive imagination,' a fellow writer said to me. 'We're creatives. So we can imagine all sorts, including our partner shagging someone else.' Heck, yes. I script lines, lingering looks, romantic settings for what are platonic coffees... Previously, I would have laid that emotion on my partner, sat back, folded my arms, and waited for them to fix it for me. *I'm jealous. Fix me.* But these days, I know: my irrational jealousy isn't for them to hold. It's mine to hold. To lug around while I run, cry, yell, write. Until it's gone. (And it *did* go, after a few days).

When emotions don't go, don't dissipate, that's when I reach out, whether to a loved one or for professional help. But I reserve my reach-outs for that which I can't solve or soothe myself. I rarely take my emotion to the person I feel it about because it's so rarely true. 'I feel like you're neglecting me': they're just busy, peach. 'I feel like you don't love me any more': there's no real evidence for that, is there?

The Buddhists think sitting through discomfort is the flame in which we are forged. That the only way out is through. And I've found that learning to go *through,* without external help, is unbelievably empowering.

THE TERRIBLE TWINS:
BOOZE & COCAINE

INT. LIVING ROOM. HIGHGATE. WITCHING HOUR

CATHERINE GRAY and her superior, BOSS, have been drinking their tits off in Soho and doing 'karaoke' (read: 'tuneless yelling', which could be used to torture war criminals).

Now, they are drinking more at BOSS's fancy townhouse, because they definitely haven't had enough already. BOSS pads across a silk-threaded rug to slide an ornamental box, the colour of duck eggs, off a shelf. Holy mackerel, does everything here look like it cost a thousand pounds.

BOSS opens the box. Pearls, rose gold and opals push their way out of their compartments, tangling around each other like bodies at a deluxe jewellery orgy.

BOSS: *'Want some?'*

She's popped open a secret drawer; a hidden drug dungeon, in which there's at least three grams of cocaine, plus a tiny silver shovel that looks like something a royal Sylvanian Family's butler would use to shovel snow off the palace's driveway.

CATHERINE: *'Ummm, I dunno. I'm not very good at doing coke. I've only done it about five times. The last time, I cried the entire next day.'*

BOSS: *'It's really good stuff.'*

CATHERINE: *'OK, can you show me how?'*

BOSS plucks a pre-rolled fifty pound note from a compartment above. She demonstrates. CATHERINE follows suit.

ONE HOUR LATER:

CATHERINE and BOSS are lying in BOSS's bed.

CATHERINE: 'I think you're my best friend.'

BOSS sighs, as if to say: amateur.

BOSS: 'It's just the coke; it makes you think you love people when you don't.'

There's a pause.

CATHERINE: 'No, really. You're my best friend. Can we spoon?'

BOSS: 'No, Cath. Go to sleep.'

***

It gets better. The next morning, hanging, I ask BOSS, 'Do we *have* to go into work? I mean, can't we just skip today?' Which was the equivalent of asking the tax man if you *have* to declare all your income. I mean, can't I just skip some? Like, the income I got in cash? That's OK, right?

I only did cocaine around fifteen times, total, but on the final time I did it, I swore to never do so again. I felt its cobra-like grip tighten. The urge for more the next time I drank. And it was an urge that felt even more demonic, even more chilling than the mania I had for more booze.

I wasn't imagining it. A 2015 study (among others) has shown that when you drink, your cocaine crave spikes. 'On average, craving peaked 15 minutes following drink completion,' the study said. Yikes.

Also, I'm really glad I never got too into cocaine since I've now been told this *time and time again*. Heavy drinkers use cocaine in order to fix up, look sharp and drink more. Say what? Crikey, am I glad I didn't know that. Because had I done, I would have likely shovelled coke up my nose with that Sylvanian butler's shovel on a regular basis.

'Interestingly, when in the Nineties the Icelandic government passed a law to allow 24-hour drinking, there was subsequently an increase in amphetamine use,' says Professor Nutt. Like coke.

'Cocaine while drinking may feel like a "sharpener", but it's more that you're now sedated but also wide awake,' says Dr Judith Grisel. 'You're drunk but alert, simultaneously.'

And – off you go – like a coked-up Roadrunner. 'You can now go longer into the night because you've got a stimulant on board,' she says. 'It's the same upper + downer effect of speedballs (heroin and cocaine), whereby you have the sedating opiate, alongside the arousing cocaine.'

Cocaine disables the natural brakes of a) visible drunkenness, meaning your mates/the bar cuts you off; b) maximum drunkenness, meaning you can no longer summon the wherewithal to locate more booze, even if you were able to obtain it; c) ~~falling asleep~~ passing out.

Those brakes are there for a bloody good reason. They're there to stop your drunk car from ploughing bumper-first into a tree.

In fact, the terrible twins of coke and booze combine to form an entirely new animal. 'Cocaine and alcohol work together in the body to produce a new chemical called cocaethylene (CE),' says Professor David Nutt. 'CE is a longer-acting form of cocaine that hangs around in the body for hours rather than minutes.' Making it more toxic to the heart.

More good news coming atcha. 'The duo also makes cocaine more lethal,' says Dr Grisel. 'Evidence shows that if you have alcohol on board already, and you then take cocaine, you're more likely to die than you would from cocaine alone. This combination augments addiction because drinking has a natural limiting barrier,' adds Dr Grisel. 'Cocaine is a way to party even more, after this natural barrier should have stopped you. It's very dangerous in that respect.'

What you have after a liberal dusting of cocaine is a car with no brakes. An equally fuckfaced person, but one who is now no longer sleepy. Instead they're wild-eyed, berserk, bouncin' and hungry for much more chaos. Chaos that could easily cost £200 in one night. And will involve mixing with the henchpeople of drug lords. Or drug lords themselves.

GREAT.

It's like the illegal equivalent of the vodka Red Bull trend that swept the nation in the late Nineties, because on cocaine, you're so awake at 2am that your eyes are on stalks, like a Ren & Stimpy character, yet your logical faculties shut down somewhere around 10pm.

Regular Drunk You would be slumbering on the sofa of this house party right now, despite the bass making the sofa vibrate like a Power Plate. But Coked 'n' Drunk You is now suggesting that you dial for more drugs and hollering for a game of strip poker, when you all have to be at work in six tiny hours.

Honestly, I think if I'd discovered cocaine's sharpening powers and had wielded the financial wherewithal to sustain a blow habit, I'd probably be dead by now. So for those of you who have managed to/are currently kicking a terrible twin habit of both booze and coke, I not only tip my hat to you, I would like to send you an entire millinery of doffed hats. R-E-S-P-E-C-T.

I'm going to hand over now to some readers who found themselves hijacked by the terrible twins, so they can tell us more about what that was like.

***

TERRIBLE TWINS GROUP-SHARE

'Cocaine just bought me time to drink more and eventually do a lot of things I normally wouldn't. I thought no one knew I was sneaking off to do coke; now I'm sober I'm not sure how anyone wouldn't know. I quit both. If I ever started on one again, I know it would definitely end up being the two.'

Scarlett

'Beer and gear is massive with men and football. You become a slave to the toilet cubicle. I can't tell you how many times I've stood in a cubicle waiting for a hand-dryer to be used, so that I could sniff the gear without suspicion. It was easy to quit coke after I quit drinking. Weirdly though, I still have vivid dreams about doing coke, probably because it releases more dopamine in the brain.'

Sam

'It was only after I knocked cocaine on the head that I realised it had enabled me to be a drinking machine. I could drink for days without going into blackout. Once cocaine was gone – BAM! Alcohol came to the fore as the real issue. I realised the quantities I was drinking were enough to sedate an elephant. I quit cocaine fairly easily by moving to a new city and trying hard not to make any, ahem, connections. Alcohol, however, was on every street corner.'

Caitlin

'I would go to a bar with an intention of a few pints and definitely no cocaine. I would easily refuse coke up until pint three, but after pint four I was like "go on then". Come 6am in the morning you're in someone's kitchen talking absolute shite to people you hardly know. My problem was working in the offshore industry, doing shifts, and having two weeks off, which became like a giant Friday night after a working week.'

Darren

'I don't ever crave cocaine until I've had the tiniest lick of alcohol. After which, I'll do anything to get it. I associated cocaine with having such a great time, but it's only good for 10 minutes. Then the rest of the time is spent obsessing about doing more coke. The only way to stop is to force sleep, which never works; you end up awake for days. Nightmare.'

Molly

'I didn't drink without cocaine, and I didn't do coke without drink. Without the drink, coke was intense and gave me too much anxiety; without the coke, alcohol made me feel sloppy and depressed. I would get obliterated with the knowledge that cocaine would be there to level me out. However, a multitude of messes were created by the mix of lost inhibitions (alcohol) and "I can do whatever the hell I please!" confidence (cocaine). I was sexually assaulted during a binge, crashed my car (was luckily unscathed), woke up in many a stranger's bed and got into a lot of debt. An episode of psychosis forced me into getting clean: a very scary time I am now so grateful for.'

Luna

'Cocaine lies to you. It makes you believe you're completely sober and in control, when the reality is very far from that. I would routinely be ordering drugs before I'd even finished my first glass of wine.'

Harpreet

'I would hide my cocaine use, so alcohol was my "show" and it allowed me to drink less but still feel buzzed. The coke became a hangover cure; I was using it at work just to stay level. In recovery, my cravings for coke have been worse than the alcohol cravings. The comedown and withdrawal from coke was hell. But I quit both at the same time, so it's hard to say which was worse. I'm fricking glad coke is illegal, though!'

Zoe

'When drunk I would go looking for cocaine to lift my mood and keep me awake so that I could keep drinking. The result was hyperactive, highly sexualised behaviour. And complete oversharing of my most private experiences. In short – I became an utter arsehole, but thought I was the absolute business.'

Georgina

'Coming down off both is like that tummy flip when you've done something really wrong – but it lasts for five days. It's relentless. I'm so glad I never have to go through that again.'

Keira

STONE COLD VS SUNSHINE WARM DOG SITTING

It's been said so many times before, but that's because it's true. Drinking turns us into hangdog detectives, who have to bloodhound around for clues the morning after as to what the hell happened.

I know people who have gone and inspected the bumper of their car for evidence of hair and blood (one spine-chilling morning for an American friend involved finding both; she later had a flashback of hitting a deer), after a blacked-out drive home.

Or we have to steel ourselves (please no) as we check our call logs, text history and sent emails. I have another friend who would delete all of her drunken message chains, as if to protect her sober self from the messaging of her drunk self.

The worst detective morning I have ever experienced? The morning I thought I'd killed a dog.

STONE COLD DRUNK DOG SITTING

APRIL 2013

10am: I am wrenched awake, rudely, by someone singing downstairs. So bloody early! The banging that accompanies it suggests they're cleaning windows or somesuch wholesome activity. 'I hope you fall out of the window,' I think, heaping medieval curses upon their chirpy head.

I lie on my side, eyes closed, willing myself to go back to sleep, as I always tell myself more sleep will nix the hangover. I finally give up and drag my eyes open. Across the yellowing vintage bedspread throw I find myself eye-to-eye with a flea. Hopping around impishly. I squash it with my finger and its blood (my blood, no doubt) leaves a red star on the bedspread that desperately needs a wash anyway.

It's from my boyfriend's Jack Russell. The flea, I mean. Not me. I call out to the dog, who I allow to sleep with me, mainly for my comfort, not his, hence the hopping bedfellow. 'Smudge. SMUDGE!' Where the chuff is Smudge? I heave myself up and sway to the kitchen.

Smudge isn't in the living room, or the kitchen, or the spare room. I find his lead. But no Smudge. Panic starts to rise in my throat, like heartburn. I scour my memory of last night.

I took Smudge to a wine bar down the road, in this sleepy riverside village that I moved to in the hope its lack of nightlife would inhibit my drinking. It hasn't. I just drink at home more. (I later find out they call this a 'geographical fix' where you move to a place, in the hope it will un-break your drinking)

I remember Smudge looking up at me, with big chocolate eyes, whimpering slightly, begging to leave this godforsaken place where people just got louder and clumsier, as my friend Emma and I drank wine after wine.

I remember perching him on my lap at the bar while I continued talking with strangers long after Emma had left. I remember giving him to a stranger to hold while I went to the loo. I remember another stranger trying to show himself into the loo with me, under the misapprehension I was up for it, and me pushing him out.

And then – nothing. I don't remember leaving the bar, or getting home with Smudge, or whether I left with Smudge, or whether the stranger still had Smudge, or whether Smudge got run over and I wept and then detached his lead from his cold crushed body.

For a full half hour, I am convinced that I have killed Smudge, somehow. I cry and cry. And then my phone, grubby with fingerprints and cigarette ash, vibrates into life. It's my boyfriend, calling from his weekend away.

'*My mum just called*,' *he says. '*She's just got home from her sister's. Did you drop Smudge at hers last night? He's peed on the wallpaper. Why'd you do that?*'*

***

It seems that in some bizarre attempt to protect Smudge from my drunken alter ego, I used the spare key I have for his mum's place to drop him there, when I was completely off my tits. I have absolutely no recollection.

Smudge lives on, despite me. But the memory of having nearly killed him, by being wasted and in charge of a helpless animal with zero road sense, is one of my hundred-strong tiny rock bottoms. Smudge is still devoted to me afterwards (as dogs usually are despite maltreatment) but I notice a newfound quiver when I pick him up.

And every time he quivers in my arms, I think – I was meant to protect you and I didn't. I'm sorry buddy.

SUNSHINE WARM SOBER DOG SITTING

NOVEMBER 2020

I now dog sit a total of six dogs, either for full fortnights or the odd evening.

Barney and Ruby the Cocker Spaniels, Floyd the Becapoo (Bedlington meets Cavapoo. Floyd is a law unto himself), Pina the Greek rescue dog, Pablo the working Cocker, Archie the Miniature Dachshund... oh, and two cats – Cyril and Lola.

I have the keys for two other people's houses hanging on my key hook. I am trusted with people's houses as well as their cherished fam-imals (yep, I went there).

In fact, I finally feel ready for my own. And with that, I make plans for a puppy. I know I don't mind picking up poo, or walking at 6am if needs be, or giving endless cuddles to the trembling, or throwing a ball 39 times. I have even been known to rub cream into a dog's anus because he had a rash.

I now know that I will make an excellent dog parent. And after that? Who knows? I'm open-minded. I can finally trust myself, as well as be trusted by others, to do what parenting requires: unconditional love + nurturing.

And of course, I now know I can do the third central tenet of parenting – bums.

THE NINE THINGS I'VE
LEARNED ABOUT LOVING
BOOZEHOUNDS

It made sense that when I was still getting spangled, the lion's share of my friends could handle their liquor. Moderate drinkers backed away from me slowly, groping behind them for a wooden stake and holy water, thinking *you'll be the death of me. Begone!*

Whereas teetotallers? Forgetaboutit. Because I was a wanker to teetotallers. I once said to a potential buddy, 'Oh no, you're teetotal?! What a shame, for a moment there I thought we could be friends.'

So, I surrounded myself with other big drinkers, on the whole. But now I'm sober, and what's peculiar is that I still gravitate towards the 'night seekers'. The party animals. Most of the friends I've made in the past seven years are either ex- or current hellraisers.

Many are retired, but many are still chasing the night to the very end, still helter skelter after the rabbit with the pocket watch; down, down, down the rabbit hole they go, where they'll end up, nobody knows.

Why is this? Simple. Because I'm like them, and *I like them*, whether they're on my side of the curtain now or not. This does, of course, throw up some interesting challenges. Dilemmas. And lessons.

1. DRINKERS FEEL JUDGED BY ME

It doesn't matter how many times I repeat, 'I drank my face off for 21 years, I'm the last one to judge'. They feel judged. Just as I did, when I drank.

I was recently walking past a couple of friends who were sitting on a balcony 30 feet away. I waved enthusiastically, like the village idiot. They waved back and hollered down, 'This is a soft drink!', gesturing to a pitcher of icy liquid sitting between them. I gave them a thumbs up, but what I really wanted to yell back was, 'So what? I don't care!'

It's not my business – or concern – what's in their glass. You do you, boo.

2. THERE'S A DISCONNECT BETWEEN PUBLIC/ PRIVATE

'How terrible that you can't drink wine!' one now-friend barked at me across a table when we first met. Later, she would tell me that she wished she could stop drinking wine because it makes *her* feel terrible.

As much as drink-pushing like this makes me bristle, especially when it's done to the newborn sober, I now dig deep for compassion. Because I've been that drink-pusher. I think hard on the time I toppled a colleague's quit by heckling her until she capsized into a Chenin Blanc. I remember the time I cattily described a teetotaller dancing as awkward anathema: 'like a giraffe trying to ice skate'. *She* didn't look uncomfortable but she made *me* uncomfortable. It's astounding, really, how many sober people are reformed drink-pushers.

I now accept that there will be that disconnect between what people say to me in private and what they say as a public heckle. I remember that here in the brightly lit bar, they're sniding me with 'well *you're no fun*', but back in their dimly lit home, they're likely the ones *no longer having fun* in their drinking.

And so – compassion.

3. WORRY IS FUTILE

Worrying about someone feels like an activity. It feels like a protection charm, like maybe it will hang a talisman around their neck, protecting them from harm. But sadly, it does no such thing. My father used to say that worry is a meditation on 'shit that could go wrong'. And it is. It's an irresistibly futile meditation on potential catastrophe. Which does absolutely zip to prevent it.

You can't change *them*. All you can do is change how you *react to them*. Tiptoeing downstairs after they've retired to snuff out the candles they tend to leave burning. Putting them in the recovery position, if they've passed out. Limiting your contact with them when they're half in the bag.

I've been known to drag furniture across my doorway when living in a houseshare with a heavy drinker. I've lain in bed, hearing strange men being shown into the living room at 3am. ('But they're from Chelsea!' my housemate said the next day, as if a posh postcode inoculates someone from being a psychopath). I get it, of course. When you're drunk, bringing strangers (new friends!) home seems fun. When you're sober, it seems insane.

I couldn't change her. I could, however, block my doorway. So I did.

4. EX-DRINKERS MAKE EXCELLENT HANGOVER ALLIES

I don't enable. I no longer pretend to love watching my friends get blasted for six hours. I won't buy a wasted friend another drink, accompany them to da (dodgy) club, or hang around once I've answered the same question three times.

What I will do is buy them a tea instead, get them some food, offer to see them home in my taxi, or kindly explain that we've already had this conversation, and maybe it's now time for me to bounce.

But come the next day, I am *the most* sympathetic and helpful hangover ally. I take loved ones smoothies in bed. I scratch their backs and give them ibuprofen. I talk slowly, move slowly. Make them a pepper and mushroom frittata, if they can stomach it. I know about the darkness they find themselves enveloped in. I want to soften it, if I can. Bring a little light into the room.

My friends know now that I won't help them into their hangover, but I will help them out of it.

5. THE SUBTEXT TO THE MORNING-AFTER TEXT

I know about the morning-after text. It's those chirpy incidentals I sent out to my mates. 'Whoa, what about last night hey?! I woke up with a Happy Meal toy in my hand. I'm guessing we went to Maccy Ds? Are we now barred for life?!'

It seemed straightforward to them. A matter-of-fact reminisce about the night before. But I would sit on tenterhooks, swinging on suspense, until they replied. When I would then snatch my phone up, half-relieved, half-dreading, to read the verdict. Because what I was really saying in that morning-after text was: 'I've woken up and I'm frightened. I don't remember. Are we OK?'

I know about the subtext. So I always respond to 'Are we OK?' chirrups quickly and kindly.

6. WHAT HANGOVER DENYING MEANS

I used to do this, didn't (or don't) you? Think that if I admitted to dying inside from a hangover, that somebody would stop my drinking. That the drinking police would show up and snatch away my 'fun'. I would sit there, clearly hanging, and claim to be feeling tickety-boo.

There's a strange irony in the truth that the person most likely to 'fess up to feeling ransacked, wrecked and ravaged by a hangover –

who will sit there looking pale and haunted rather than trying to plaster it over with bravado, make-up or more booze – is probably the one with the better relationship with alcohol.

The kindest thing to do is not 'out' them. I once met a friend on the street who had a monstrous hangover. I knew because I'd seen the Instagram stories from 2am. She was shaking like a chihuahua. 'I'm so nervous about my driving lesson,' she claimed. I knew. I said nothing.

7. RADICAL HONESTY VS TOUGH LOVE

If my barfly friends ask me 'How bad was I?', 'Do I need to apologise to so-and-so?' or 'What did I say?' I will tell them. I won't roll that turd in glitter. As, looking back, I wish others hadn't sugared what they told me.

I don't believe in tough love. I've been on the receiving end of it and it did nothing useful, other than dragging my self-esteem, which was already in the gutter, down into the sewer.

But what has had a profound effect on me has been radical honesty. I once bemoaned to my best mate that I was tired of people calling me Booze Hag and Bad Santa and suchlike. 'Why can't they see all the other things about me?' I cried. 'Like the running, the writing, the... the... y'know, the other *things*?' (I'd run out of things because my main hobby was drinking).

With a world-weary mix of grit and grace, she told me, 'If you want them to see something different, show them something different.' It turned an important cog in my head.

Disclaimer: *they* need to bring their drinking up. So, wait. And then: 'What am I like when I'm drunk?' they might ask. This is your cue to take their hand and tell them the truth. 'I actually prefer you when you're sober. That's when you're your best self. Sober You is an absolute legend.'

8. INTERVENTIONS GENERALLY DON'T WORK

I'm frequently asked, 'What can I do to help my sister/brother/ mother/best mate/partner get sober?' With the exception of the aforementioned radical honesty, my answer is always, 'Unless they've asked you for help, alas my peach, you can do nothing.' Zip. Zilch. Nada.

It's heartbreaking but mostly true, in my opinion. You can lead someone to sobriety, but you can't make them partake. Interventions can get people into treatment, yes, but they often push them into treatment they're not ready for, meaning they start a dispiriting quit–relapse–quit–relapse grind.

The genesis of a realisation is often created within the drinker with more of a whimper than a bang. I had plenty of dramatic drunken 'bottoms'. People watching on must've thought: surely *this* will be the moment she realises. Surely she can't *not* now.

Was it when I chipped my front tooth by falling into a door after my birthday party?

Or the Friday morning I woke up in a claw-foot bathtub in a five-star hotel in Soho, to regard two people snoring in bed, neither of whom I knew (I did a mad dash around Topshop at 9am to buy new clothes to wear to work, given mine were pock-marked with red wine)? Or was it the time I was found unconscious on our doorstep by my then-boyfriend?

Nope, it was none of that. When no realisation arrives – despite the drinker being clobbered with the consequences of drinking – onlookers tend to assume it never will. Meanwhile, it's actually invisibly assembling itself within the drinker. But nobody – and nothing – can truly expedite that.

My mum and dad tried to stage an intervention on me once. It was January 2013. They sent me handwritten letters, separately, to arrive the same day. They both said they thought I should stop drinking.

I ripped them up. I was furious. I wasn't ready, and I wouldn't *be ready* until I asked for help later that same year. It couldn't be rushed. If anything, I think this joint intervention probably only served to delay my asking for help. *I'll show them*, I thought, digging my heels in deeper.

There's no such thing as a magical phrase that can spark a spontaneous quit. *Oh, you're right, I never thought about it that way!* Nor is there a rehab on earth that can make someone stay sober after they leave, unless they entered the doors with a tiny sliver of 'sick and tired of being sick and tired'. There just isn't.

9. HELP, IF THEY ASK. BUT DETACH FROM THE OUTCOME

If they ask for help, hooray! This is your time to shine. Give them books, talk it out, offer to go with them to a sober meet (of any flavour), watch documentaries together, send them links to podcasts and blogs you think they'll like.

But know this. Ultimately, when it comes to crunch time, the only person who can help them, is them. As sobriety author Laura McKowen says, 'We can't do this alone, but only we can do it.' Never a truer word spoken.

I've been asked by dozens of loved ones to help them quit. I have helped. While detaching myself from their outcome. Because the outcome is theirs to hold, not mine. I can't do it for them, much as I'd love to be able to.

And nor can you, as much as you would love to. Attaching to things we cannot control is a fast lane to madness. Do what you can and then – step back.

'Not my circus, not my monkeys'
Unknown

WHEN YOU NEED TO WALK

Sometimes your only option is to walk. If you can't even *see* the end of your tether, let alone shimmy back up it.

At four years sober, some distant drinking buddies had indeed fallen away, but in general, I had the exact same close friends as I'd had as a drinker. I wore 'same friends!' like a badge of pride.

Only, I had changed enormously. You probably have too, if you're on this sober path. Nowadays, four-fifths of my close friends *are* still the same, but I have had to let some friendships go. Because we not only changed; we changed in different directions.

There was the friend who brought bags of MDMA to parties, encouraging me to have some to 'loosen up'. The friend who invited me to her birthday bash, then uninvited me because 'we're going to be getting lashed'. And the friend who I endured years of strife with, who once savagely told me that she'd *never be as bad as I was*, even though she was already drinking more than I ever had.

With all three of these friendships, I felt like a happy hypocrite for flinching whenever one used my favourite hand-painted teacup as an ashtray, because *hadn't I done the exact same thing?!* I would walk their dog, repeatedly, while they slept until 1pm. Get in the car with them when they were drink-driving. Keep my cool when they pinned me in a corner for a wild-eyed political rant after a bottle-and-a-half. Apologise to the taxi driver on their behalf, for their accusations of him taking 'the long way'.

I trudged along in these three friendships for three, five and six years after getting sober, telling myself it was karma; a price I felt I should pay. Who did I think I was, getting annoyed with *them*, when I'd once *been* them? They were just the old me! This was how my loved ones had felt *about me*, right? Right.

Until, I just couldn't any more. Watching the addiction dig its claws in was too disempowering, saddening and frustrating. We had nothing in common any more. I couldn't watch between my fingers any more. Even though I'd once been them.

You don't have to watch either. You can disengage. If you've truly had enough. It's not hypocrisy to detach with love. Three things can be true at once:

1. I love you

2. I empathise

3. I can no longer be around you.

UNREPORTED BENEFIT OF SOBRIETY #117: HIGHER FERTILITY

I was never sure I wanted children. And then my ovaries woke up when I turned 39. Thanks, ovaries. A little tardy there, dontchathink. You could've told me sooner, buddies.

Interestingly, this awakening happened the same year I finally became financially secure. No coincidence, I wager. Who knows if I'll be able to have biological children. My research shows that the fertility nosedive between 35 and 40 is much overstated, so I may well be able to. And if I can't, thankfully I'm open to the myriad other options: adoption, egg donation, surrogacy, a fur family.

When my ovaries woke up, I discovered something fascinating. Those who are sober – or who drink very little – are giving their fertility the best fighting chance. Research suggests that teetotallers and light drinkers tend to be more fertile than regular drinkers.

One Danish study analysed 6,120 women aged 21 to 45 over a time span of nine years. The women kept detailed drinking diaries throughout. Seven in ten of them conceived. When they analysed the drinking diaries, the researchers discovered that a 250ml glass of wine a day cut the chances of conception by 18 per cent. Eighteen per cent!

Other studies showed that even light drinking had an impact. Another Danish study looked at 430 couples and concluded that if the woman drank five – or fewer – drinks a week, it led to reduced fertility.

Meanwhile, a Harvard study analysed 4,729 IVF cycles. Refreshingly, this study looked at both male and female intake of alcohol (seems *truly bizarre* that the others didn't, as if conception is purely a female issue?!).

This study found that when both partners drank six or more units per week, the odds of having a live baby were 21 per cent lower than the couples who drank less. In laymen's terms, this means that if a couple split just over *a bottle of wine a week*, they were a fifth less likely to conceive. Bonkers.

'If you are going to have IVF, my recommendation would be that it makes sense to avoid alcohol altogether, from three months beforehand,' said Tony Rutherford, chairman of the British Fertility Society, in a *Guardian* piece reporting on the findings.

Interesting, hey? And what's even more interesting is that, before this discovery dig, I'd never heard even a whisper that drinking could slash your chances of conceiving. Had you? And yet, some of these studies date back 20 years. *Le sigh*. It's just another example of the hushed-up harms of drinking.

BURNING QUESTION:
IS ADDICTION A DISEASE?

Dr David Nutt says: 'Yes, addiction is a disease. It impairs function, shortens life and affects work and family abilities. It has a known cause (see page 165) and there are treatments (12 step and so on) that work in some people.'

Dr Marc Lewis says: 'No. That's why I wrote a whole book (*The Biology of Desire*) subtitled *Why Addiction is Not a Disease*. It's not a brain disease, however it does, of course, change the brain.

The phenomenon of synaptic configurations means that with any recurring, highly motivated activity, you're going to get synaptic "superhighways" – what you would call motorways in Britain – that carry most of the brain's traffic. Those superhighways are the best way to think about addiction.

Synaptic superhighways are the brain's way of streamlining. This neural adaptation is how we become an expert in something specific: say a neurosurgeon or concert musician. But in addiction, that streamlining – of tendencies to use an addictive substance or activity – means that other potential pathways, offshoots and detours fade. Your brain becomes like a town with one highway running through it, rather than many smaller streets.

However, we almost need to put the brain story aside, given we can't go in with neurosurgical tools and change the brain directly. So we treat addiction through interpersonal activities and methods, which over long periods of time then change the brain too.'

Dr Judith Grisel says: 'If we could define what "disease" is, that would really help. If the sign of a disease is that it's progressive and chronic, then yes, I believe it is.'

Dr Julia Lewis says: 'Technically, it's not necessarily a disease, but politically, it needs to be seen and managed as one given it physically alters the body. The chronic disease management model, developed in the US, fits well for the management of addiction. It acknowledges that it's not a case of fix and then discharge. Like asthma and diabetes, you may go through long periods where you're well, but then brief spurts where you need support. It needs low-key background management. If things go belly up, you need to be able to access the professionals easily and quickly. Therefore the "disease management" model is not a *perfect* pigeonhole for addiction, but it's the best place to put it.'

ANXIETY SOOTHING SUPERSIZED

Yes, I realise the acronym of this chapter is ASS. That's OK with me.

Yesterday my friend Amanda saw me walk past at 11am when she was brunching and later told me: 'You looked so serene. Like you'd just spent the morning drinking lemony water, doing yoga and meditating.'

'Ha,' I said. 'If only you knew.'

That morning my insides had resembled Edvard Munch's *The Scream*, despite my outsides resembling Snow White.

There is a whopping link between GAD (generalized anxiety disorder) and big drinking. Given incidence of addicted drinking in those with social anxiety is pegged at around 20 per cent, that means anxious bears are around twice as likely to become hooked.

Alcohol acts as an anxiety eraser. 'It removes an adverse state,' says psychologist and neuroscientist Dr Judith Grisel. 'If you're using it to medicate anxiety, you'll like it because it removes the anxiety. It's a sedative, after all, and it reduces inhibitions. Those *not* prone to anxiety don't like it as much. They're more likely to dislike the sloppy feeling, or their words slurring. But if you're anxious, you enjoy that blur. It becomes your antidote to anxiety.'

Anyone who's gotten, or is getting, sober will know this. Us anxious bears have minds that never shut the hell up. It's like having a loquacious toddler, one prone to catastrophizing and asking absurd questions, running around inside our brains. We used the booze to achieve narcoleptic nothingness, and now that we don't use it, the rabbiting toddler is trying to drive us quite mad.

1. FINDING THE ANTI-CHATTER

People find their anti-chatter in various ways. It's entirely individual as to what stills your mind, quietens it, gives it an outlet.

Try this thought experiment. It helps me. I now think of anxiety as energy, or *Alice in Wonderland*-esque 'muchness'. That nervous thrum can either sit in our tanks, souring into anxiety, or be spent elsewhere. We can use it to keep our houses shipshape, to send ten emails in ten minutes, to write poetry, wild swim or make homemade cards with watercolour pens.

The 'muchness' needs a place to go. So I give it one. Lately, I've fallen in love with the laser-focused concentration of bouldering. When you're on a climbing wall five metres up with no ropes, believe me, you're not thinking about anything else but how to *not fall off the wall.* Friends of mine take their meditation cushion and timer everywhere. But I tend to find my finest stillness of mind in movement.

2. SCUBA GEAR IN A STORM

What about when you can't go for a run, or meditate, or clean, or write your anxiety away? When it's been summoned by being seated in the restaurant, the swish of a lift shutting, or the click of a meeting-room door. You feel pinned in place, helplessly stuck, while elemental titans whip around you.

Welcome to the head-storm. Oh, cruel irony: the more you fight the roar, the more intense the experience gets.

How do you learn to trust that your heart will not stop, your lungs will not fail and you will not projectile vomit all over the train/dinner/meeting-room table? How do you learn to trust that everything will be OK, even when it feels terrifically like it *will not*?

'We all know people who are "everyday Buddhas"', says neuropsychologist Dr Rick Hanson. 'Who, despite it all, sustain an unshakeable core of resilient kindness and wellbeing.'

They confound us; we wonder how they do it. Dr Hanson says it's deceptively simple. 'Repeated internalisation of beneficial experiences'. Or, in other words, by tattooing the positive of life onto our brains. 'By installing the residues of beneficial experiences, we literally create lasting physical changes in our nervous system,' Dr Hanson reveals.

He likens the resulting untouchable core of inner peace as like having scuba-diving gear in a stormy ocean. 'On the surface, colossal waves could be crashing,' he says. 'Yet, just 15 metres below the surface, you can find calm and strength, if you have the gear to get there, to drop down.' That's what those people have, and boy, do we all want a piece of that.

The way into it is via the 'repeated beneficial' clocking that Dr Hanson mentions. If you never notice when the weather is good, you'll only notice when the weather is bad. When all is OK, truly feeling that, internalising that, appreciating that, can help you trust that on the other side of this growling gale, it will be OK once more. Because OK is the default.

3. CAFFEINATED ANXIETY

I halved my caffeine during this year and – shocker – became half as anxious. Who knew? What's that you say? You ALL knew? But have you actually acted upon it? Because I too knew that, but I didn't do a rat's ass about it. For years.

Caffeine stimulates anxiety because the body interprets it as such. 'The natural effects of caffeine stimulate a host of sensations, such as your heart beating faster, your body heating up, your breathing rate increasing – all things that mimic anxiety,' Dr Susan Bowling told *Health* magazine. 'Psychologically, it's difficult for your mind to recognize that this is not anxiety because it feels the same.'

4. RADIATING LOVING-KINDNESS

Anxiety is essentially narcissistic. It's just that, instead of the 'me, me, me' voice saying 'I'm so great', it says 'I'm so weird'. It consistently negs us for feeling jittery about the elementary act of going for lunch ('what's wrong with you?!') like an arch *Mean Girl*. It tells us that everyone else in the restaurant or tube carriage is also side-eyeing us and thinking we're weird, when the reality is they've probably barely noticed us. It's the conviction that we're the oddball centre of the universe.

Neuroscientist Chris Frith says the brain performs a sleight of hand, making us believe that we're the 'actor at the centre of the world'. For many people, this may feel quite fun, being centre stage in their own personal drama, but for anxious people, it's the seventh circle of 'feeling intensely seen' hell. It's a headfuck.

One way to snap out of it is by slipping on an invisibility cloak and dropping down from centre stage into the audience. How? By swivelling attention entirely to other people. And sending them some loving kindness.

I learned this from meditation app *Buddhify*, which took it from traditional Buddhism. 'May you be well, may you be happy,' I think, as I stare at the stranger on the tube, sending them a Care Bear rainbow of goodwill. Sometimes I even architect a life around them, as if I'm playing *The Sims*, mind-building where they might live, imagining what they like to do when they get home, whether their bedroom is pin-neat or adolescent-messy.

Then I choose another person and rainbow-vibe them. I feel invisible to myself, for a blissful moment. I've remembered I'm not the oddball centre of a melodrama set in a train carriage.

5. FEEL FREE TO *NOT* DO IT

If something sends you into an anxious tailspin, and you don't have to do it, feel free to not bloody do it. I've done pretty much everything I ever did drunk as a sober now, with one exception; karaoke. When I told my witty, wry publisher about this, she kidded that the book publication party for my first book was going to be 'karaoke-themed, and the finale will be you singing a song'.

I've only attempted to do it once. I got all the way to the train station. When it came to exiting the train station and going to the karaoke bar, I couldn't do it. I was four years sober, and I couldn't do it. So, I didn't. I texted my organiser friend – sober too, so *of course* she understood – and went home instead.

It's OK if you never do sober karaoke. Nobody said we have to do everything as a sober that we did as a drinker. Given my singing voice, I think of my abstaining from karaoke as a community service.

III: YEAR SEVEN

YEAR SEVEN: ASKING FOR WHAT WE NEED

In this year, I realise: I am hopeless at asking for what I need. I don't exactly know why. I only know that I've been conditioned out of it.

Maybe because I'm a woman and womxn are traditionally taught to orbit the needs of others. Maybe because I spent years working on magazines where you are constantly told you are lucky to have your job, and anything less than genuflecting to superiors is regarded as 'an attitude'.

While drunk, I shouted my needs. I insisted upon them. 'More drinks!' I would yell, a thirsty harpy. 'Gimme cigarette!' I would encroach, of utter strangers. I was a need-barking brat. When I get sober, I learn to give more than I get.

New me! My go-to when I'm feeling down becomes doing something kind for someone else. Indeed, there's a persuasive hub of research to show that doing something for someone else – 'kindfulness' – works better than doing something for ourselves. A 2008 study found that, when people spent a surprise windfall on others, they felt happier than when they spent it on themselves.

The 'helper's high' we get from altruism could even potentially soften withdrawal (this is entirely my speculation) given brain scans show that kind acts ding-a-ling delightfully through the striatum (not my speculation: a fact), the same reward-obsessed part of the brain that generates addiction. Reward: replaced.

So, giving is important. Only thing is, I took it too far. I gave too much of myself away. I started thinking that my needs didn't matter and I must defer to what others wanted, needed, asked of me, in order to retain my newfound silk sash of 'Good Girl'. On cue, I smiled, postured, agreed and twirled my metaphorical baton. *Please forgive me!* I twirled. *I'll do anything you want!*

There was one defining moment when I realised how much I'd sidelined my own needs.

NEEDS #1

My friend and I are driving home from a night out. I'm feeding my fully fledged peppermint tea addiction by pouring from a flask into a keep-cup in the car (while a passenger, I hasten to add). The teabag sticks, so I think it's nearly empty. I tip it all the way up, the teabag dislodges and VOOM: boiling water all over my leg. Instant, white-hot, smouldering pain.

My friend and I decide a trip to A&E (British ER) is a bit OTT. Don't want to cause a fuss! Terribly British. Don't want to take up space for the tiny matter of a thigh that feels like it's on actual fire.

The next day I feel faint. I go to the pharmacy to see what they recommend for this hand-sized blistered burn. The pharmacist looks at it and asks why I didn't go to A&E last night. He tells me to go straight to A&E. He practically adds 'you duh-brain' to the sentence.

I cab it there. My friend phones me while I'm in the cab. I tell her I can't make our Sunday lunch plans this afternoon; that I'm on my way to A&E.

Friend: 'Oh sweetheart! I'll come wait with you and drive you home after.'

Me: 'No need, honestly, I'm fine, you have stuff to do!'

Friend: 'I'll be there.'

Chrissake. She was going to be there. And I felt squirmy and uncomfortable about that, as if I was a lumbering burnt imposition, crashing into her Sunday afternoon.

But then, it got even better on the drive home from the hospital.

She said: 'You hungry?'

I practically woof, like a dog asked 'Sausages?'

Me: 'I'm absolutely starving, oh my gosh, yes, I had no lunch.'

Friend: 'Let's stop and get something. What do you feel like?'

Me: 'What do YOU feel like?'

Friend: 'I'm not hungry, I've eaten, so it's for you.'

Me: 'Ahhh, don't worry about it then, I'm not hungry!'

Friend: 'You literally just said you're starving, you weirdo.'

Me: 'Did I? Oh, but that was when I thought you were hungry too.'

Friend: 'But it doesn't matter that I'm not hungry. YOU'RE
hungry, so let's stop!'

I agree to us picking up a bag of chips from the least inconvenient place. Near where we would park anyway, from an eatery that's pretty rank. But the thought of her having to detour, park and wait while I go and get something I truly want to eat is just unthinkable.

When I tell my therapist this story, she wants to talk about it for a really long time. I realise that as a contrite sober, a rehabilitated harpy, I've gone too far in the other direction: I place being agreeable over what I actually need.

The Crane Wife

I tell my friend Kate about my 'needs' epiphany. Because Kate is some sort of curating genius who always sends me exactly what I need to read, when I need to read it, she sends me an essay called *The Crane Wife* (readily available online) by C.J. Hauser, which was published in the *Paris Review*.

The Crane Wife is mesmerising. It's about a woman who stuffs down her needs, rather than requesting them be met by her husband-to-be, who says he proposed because she wasn't 'annoying or needy'. Despite her appearance of non-neediness, she needs things. Of course she does. We all do.

'I hated that I needed more than this from him,' Hauser writes. 'There is nothing more humiliating to me than my own desires. Nothing that makes me hate myself more than being burdensome and less than self-sufficient.'

'Even now I hear the words as shameful,' Hauser continues. '*Thirsty. Needy.* The worst things a woman can be. Some days I still tell myself to take what is offered, because if it isn't enough, it is I who wants too much.'

Woah. As soon as I finish this essay, which has propped up a mirror to my 'Me? I don't need things!' soul, I read it again. And again. It makes me realise that, particularly in romantic relationships, I am hopeless at asking for what I need.

I exorcised Cool Girl long ago (nonchalant French chick who doesn't give a flying *putain* whether you return her text or not), but I do still sit pretty and wait for my needs to somehow manifest, even though nobody I'm dating is a frickin' mind reader.

I start realising that I respect those who ask for what they need *more* than those who don't. 'I need 15 to myself,' someone says when I'm staying at his house. I smile and say, Cool.' His motto, incidentally? 'Be valuable, not available'.

'I need to stay home and rest,' is a legitimate reason to swerve a get-together for another loved one. *She needs to stay home and rest.* Open-mouthed at what I would define in myself as 'cheek' but define in others as 'class', I wonder why I never feel able to say that myself. *I need to stay home and rest.* I practise it over and over in my head, like an incantation, but I still don't use it.

NEEDS #2

And then, as the mischievous universe is wont to do, it lobs me a curveball whereby I have to ask for what I need, or watch a fledgling romantic relationship founder.

I'm a slightly anxious attacher (previously: hysterical). Which means that if I don't hear from someone I'm dating for over 48 hours, I assume that I'm never going to hear from them again. I think things are flatlining when they're tickety-boo. I grieve relationships over and over when I'm still in them. Oh, it's *such fun*.

One week, I don't hear from the guy I'm dating for four days, so I assume he now hates me and we're no longer dating. I do the mature thing, of course. I finish it. Via text. 'It feels like you're not into this, so let's just leave it,' *whips hair and flounces away*. When his reply reveals he is utterly confounded by my melodramatic 'ending things' text, we meet up for lunch.

I've rehearsed what I'm going to say at lunch. But here's the catch, when you ask for what you need. People can say no. And if they do, you need to be willing to cut them loose. Oof.

Me: 'I'm sorry for ending things. That's not what I want.'

He nods, smiles.

Me: 'Thing is, I'm what's called an "anxious attacher", which means that I need two things to feel OK: consistency and contact.'

He shuffles in his chair.

Me: 'We don't need to talk every day or anything, but I can't handle you going dark on me for that long. I need contact most days, even if just a one-line text.'

He says something vague about that being fine, but when he's busy with work he might not be able to, yadda yadda. The conversation moves along. I feel like I've failed. We're talking about the menu now. About what the heck 'nduja is. I shift in my seat. Gird myself. I go back in.

Me: 'So, I just need to circle back to that point again. About consistency and contact.'

Him: 'Uh huh?' (looking up 'nduja on his phone)

Me: 'Thing is, if I don't get that regular contact, then that's fine, I won't be angry, but we won't be dating any more. We'll revert to being friends.'

He puts his phone down and looks at me, a little startled. And then I say something I've never said before, which was unplanned, and just so happens to be a slogan for a goliath of a beauty brand.

Me: 'I'm worth it.'

Silence. Forks clank. A swirl of tumbleweed whistles over the table.

Him: 'Yes. You are.'

He makes a point of contacting me daily from then on, if only for a ten-minute phone call. It gives me an anchor I need. Aged 40, after 22 adulting years on this planet, this is the first time I have ever directly and unapologetically asked for what I need in a relationship. Turns out, if you ask for what you need, people may just give it to you.

A few months on, this happens.

NEEDS #3

I'm in my co-working space, it's Sunday, on a week when I've worked every day. My energy candle is not only burned at both ends, it's a mere wick.

I'm reading a piece of paper when I notice that my left eye's vision has a hole in it. A burned white space where words should be. As if I'm looking into the sun.

Next, the overheard lights start to hurt. My head tightens like a contracted muscle, as if a python has wrapped itself around it. I go into a dark room, curl up into a ball and close my eyes for ten minutes. I then feel my way to the toilets and splash water in my eyes.

Half an hour later, I'm officially scared that I still can't see. (I'll later find out that this is a retinal migraine but, right now, I can't look at the computer to find this out.) I don't even think twice about what to do next. I call him.

'I need you. I can't see properly and I'm scared.'

He asks where I am. And then: 'I'm coming.'

And then, you're not going to freakin' believe what I did. I put the phone down. I'm not kidding! I didn't thank him profusely, or over-explain, or roll it in 'you're the best' glitter, or tie my request up with a ribbon of regret for putting him out.

He comes and finds me, gives me some shades, sits on the dark floor with me and gives me a long hug, then leads me out of the office by the arm. I still can't see properly, so he ushers me into the car, me wearing his Ray-Bans and my woollen sweater with pink leopards on it, like some sort of badass grandma. And then, he drives me home.

I thank him, of course. But I don't apologise for having needed his help.

***

It was nothing short of a personal revelation. If you relate to any of this, I encourage you: start asking for what you need. People may say no. But equally, they may say yes.

> 'Up until the point when I went into treatment, I'd never asked for help from anybody. I would rather not have known the answer than have to ask you for help. That's why treatment was fascinating for me. They deliberately put in your path as many things as they could that required you to ask someone else how it's done. Making a cup of coffee: There's a machine over there with all these components that you've got to put together to make a cup of coffee, and I just didn't know how. So I had to ask someone. Over and over, I had to ask for help.'
>
> Eric Clapton

STONE COLD VS SUNSHINE WARM BREAK-UPS

STONE COLD DRUNK BREAK-UP

AUGUST 2011

My boyfriend knows I'm lying to him.

The deep irony is, he thinks I'm pulling other men when insofar as I'm aware (because: blackouts), I've never cheated on him (he's one of the rare partners I'm faithful to). However, he's right about the lies.

Drinking, every relationship I have is built upon a foundation of lies. I pretend to be successful (rather than in a career tailspin), healthy (runs hangovers away twice a week), a functioning adult (reality: has moved back in with parents three times in past decade), financially capable (Bahaha. Hence the return to the nest) and kind (when tanked up, I throw words like spears).

Then they get to know me. Inevitably, when whoever-I'm-dating gets deeper inside the relationship, they begin to smell the colony of rats scampering around beneath the floorboards of the fake reality I have built for them. They start to love me less. Not more. It's topsy-turvy.

I stay up later than him to 'watch TV'. 'I'm just so hooked on this show,' I lie, hunkering deeper down into the sofa and blowing a kiss goodnight. As soon as he's safely in bed, light out, I softly close the adjoining door and creep into the kitchen to pour another glass. I stay up later not to watch TV, but to drink more.

He asks me to stop drinking, aside from at weekends. I pretend I'm not drinking, when I am. I sit in my flatshare's postage-stamp London garden, call him and swear I'm drinking tea, when I'm actually drinking cider. It's a blinking good job video calling isn't on your average phone yet.

When I put the phone down, I feel the judgement radiating from the eyes of blackened windows. I stare back at them defiantly. The truth is, there's most likely no one watching. They're busy in there, getting on with their lives, while I'm busy out here, getting drunk.

His suspicions about my cheating reach interrogation level when he hears me pick up the phone, while saying, 'Ssssh, if he hears you he'll be paranoid', to a man I'm having a cigarette with outside a bar.

He dumps me. Of course. Story of my life.

A few days later, I ask him to come over. I've been alone for the weekend, drinking to anaesthetize the split. I get all of the empty bottles out from their hiding places. I place them on the kitchen floor, spaced perfectly evenly, labels out, like a police line-up. Three bottles of wine and four beer bottles, over just two nights. I'm finally ready to tell the truth.

'That's what I've drunk,' I sob, 'over just two nights, all by myself. I have a problem and I need help.' He's the first person I've ever said this to. I tell him about the suicidal ideation too.

He stays for five minutes. Offers to pay for addiction counselling. Then he leaves; me practically on my knees, begging him not to, clutching at his jacket. We never talk again, other than over Messenger to arrange how not to bump into each other at friends' birthday parties. So much for honesty, I think. I allow this experience to drive my drinking further underground. It's another two years before I'll ask for help again.

But it wasn't the honesty that was the problem. I was asking the wrong person for help. If you want help getting out of a hole, find someone who has gotten out of the same hole themselves.

SUNSHINE WARM SOBER BREAK-UP

AUGUST 2019

My boyfriend and I have broken up. We see the best in each other but bring out the worst. After nearly a year of our tiresome fight–make up–repeat cycle, it's a mutual decision. Heartbreaking but necessary.

We decide to go on our booked French holiday regardless, as a final hurrah. The morning we are meant to leave, I start projectile vomiting. Food poisoning. Probably the only time in my life I've actually had it – rather than said I had it when I actually had wine poisoning.

I need to vacate my flat anyway, as I'd offered it to a friend visiting from Belgium. I call my ex. 'What am I gonna do?' I say. 'Hang tight,' he says. 'I'm coming to get you.'

He drives for two hours, from Hertford to Brighton, scoops the shivering, disgusting mess of me up, and drives the two hours back to his. I can't eat for the next 48 hours. When I can, he makes me toast, soup and veggie roasts, nursing me back to health. He writes me a song on his guitar. We go for short walks, once I'm up to it. He runs me baths. We cuddle and watch films.

His cat sits and stares at me, unblinking, unimpressed by my invasion, and determined to be unconquered despite having known me for 11 months. He licks his paw. If he could talk he'd say, 'When are you leaving, bitch? I thought you two had split?!'

The love between my ex and I has shapeshifted, because it had to. But it still exists, in a different form. And I know that if I need him, even now that we haven't seen each other for a year+, he'll be there for me, like a shot.

His cat? His cat wouldn't spit on me if I was on fire. He'd probably pull up a seat and eat tuna treats while watching me burn.

WHY ARE DOCTORS MORE LIKELY TO BE BIG DRINKERS?

It's a commonly peddled myth that a high IQ or higher education inoculates you against addiction. In fact, reams of research show that it's quite the opposite. Stark data shows that doctors are three times as likely to develop cirrhosis than their average patient.

Meanwhile, lawyers are another profession that sees an on-average doubled risk of alcohol addiction; likely because of similar levels of stress, trauma (especially if they work in crime), culture and long hours.

The more we earn, the more likely we are to drink hard. A 2019 NHS report found that, 'The proportion of adults usually drinking at increased or higher risk of harm was highest in higher income households for both men and women, with 35% of men and 19% of women.'

But why is medicine, in particular, so much higher in addicted drinking rates? I asked some doctors to give us an inside track on this little traversed subject.

'Medical students are the heaviest drinkers at uni'

Harry, a general medical hospital doctor says:

'It's perceived as very cool to drink at medical school. At my university, the medical students were the heaviest drinkers. For me, I ran into trouble with it not when I was dealing with seriously unwell people, but when I was working horrendous hours. I drank after night shifts because I couldn't sleep. Doctors in A&E finish four out of five shifts after 8pm and only get one in four weekends off. It's isolating. Your friends and family are at work when you wake up and are asleep when you come home. Which is why medics stick together.

I think there was a part of me that also thought I was too clever to fall into the over-drinking trap. "I know the warning signs; I'll never get that bad," I thought. But when I did get *that* bad, like when I was hungover at work, I thought, "I can't let anyone know about this." Knowing the facts doesn't protect you.

Doctors are headstrong. We're the ones who are there for the most vulnerable. We're afraid to ask for help as it can have an impact on our careers. We think, "I'll sort this out myself." It took me months to own up to my own doctor about my drinking.

My hospital knows everything now and has been very supportive. My seniors were amazing. If you can be honest and say, "This is what's happened," it's unlikely to be thrown back in your face.'

'Doctors drink to get through the trauma of the job'

Mia, an intensive care doctor says:

'After medical school, the "work hard, play hard" culture carries on. Doctors party with more senior doctors; consultants who will pay the bar tab. Gradually it becomes less acceptable to binge drink (what's funny when you're 23 isn't so funny in your 30s) so people just become more secretive.

We drink to get through the trauma of the everyday. It might be the terrible delivery of a baby. You don't say, "That was an awful cardiac arrest, I want to go home and drink chamomile tea and do yoga." The sadness lingers, so we would go out as a group to cope. You'd start the night re-hashing the trauma, asking your shift team: "Could I have done something differently?"

It's alarming how many doctors are addicted to something.

Anaesthetists have a reputation for being addicted to controlled drugs because they have easier access to them. But alcohol is more socially acceptable and drink driving doesn't always get you struck off.

The higher rates of cirrhosis can only be because of chronic alcohol intake. Being a doctor means a very disrupted lifestyle; you change jobs every six to 12 months, you often move house then too, and move away from your social support. Your new hospital gives you new friends, but they're not true friends; they're your pub mates. You've maybe lost your non-medical friends and your mum isn't around to say you look like shit. You sleep poorly, you reach for the quick fix to turn off the sadness, and there's this false self-assurance that *you're* not going to get cirrhosis because you treat those who do.

I used to party pretty hard but I chose the lucky sober path three years ago. I do find work nights out challenging. Alcohol bonds the team. You're an outsider if you don't join in. People ask me, "Are you driving?", "Why aren't you drinking?", and are surprised I've still come out. I say, "I don't have to get drunk; I'm just here for a work night out." No one ever says, "I can't believe you're a vegetarian, why've you come out for a group meal?"

I cope with the stress in different ways now. I have a tiny little garden and grow a mixture of plants in specific locations and in extreme order. Then the rest of my garden is total chaos. Which is pretty representative of intensive care.'

'I was treating patients dying of liver disease and still getting hammered every weekend'

Mark, a junior doctor says:

'It starts in medical school. I went to Imperial College, a university whose weekly sports night were so boozy it once landed itself in the *Daily Mail*. I took several friends to A&E with alcohol poisoning on different occasions during my time there. It's almost expected that you go a bit wild on nights out when you spend the rest of your time studying.

When you're let loose onto the wards as a qualified doctor, you remain unprepared to deal with the chronic stress that the job entails – most of it actually remains unrecognised and can manifest itself as a continuation of the drinking culture that many people leave behind as they get older. We tut at those who come to hospital with alcohol poisoning and drunken injuries, and then we ourselves joke about needing a drink at the end of our shift.

I recently found myself in A&E managing the airway of a man who had collapsed after a cardiac arrest while mowing the lawn. We couldn't save him. I watched his wife sob over his dead body and then I left and greeted my next patient. I didn't even stop to think that being witness to this would be traumatic for many people. That's our daily job.

I was once working on a gastroenterology ward with patients dying of liver disease and still going out and getting hammered every weekend. There's a complete disconnect between you and your patients.

When I quit alcohol last year, the vast majority of my medic friends were supportive. But a few wouldn't drop it. They'd eye-roll me: "Are you drinking again yet?" One friend, who I think was projecting his own issues with alcohol, quizzed me on, "How are you going to date? How are you going to go out?" He even asked me, word for word, "How are you going to socialise without alcohol?"

Doctors see the extremes – people who have liver disease for years and still drink, jaundiced with bloated abdomens from their failing livers. It's easy to compare yourself to that end of the spectrum and say, "That's not me". One question we're taught to ask is, "Do you drink in the morning?" And given we don't, we think our drinking isn't *that* bad.'

'It's a Venn overlap of arrogance, loneliness, self-destruction and entitlement '

Bill, a GP says:

'Doctors hardly party, but drink hard when they do. I wasn't involved in the many drinking games at medical school. My drinking escalated when I graduated and came out. It was partly celebration and making up for lost time, but also partly running away from family and responsibilities.

Loneliness is key. Junior doctors find their social lives systematically eroded by the job. We miss friends' birthdays, their weddings, Christmas with our family. But it's deeper than that too. Medics are rarely their authentic selves. We're trained to show 'disingenuous empathy', otherwise known as a 'bedside manner'. We learn how to manage people, to put on this doctor front, which means we don't show who we truly are.

I wanted to be able to exercise more, to enjoy the evenings without alcohol and to stop being a mess for my husband. So, I quit. Some people find getting sober a lonely journey, but Northern Ireland has a high proportion of teetotallers and I connected with people through One Year No Beer.

What's amazed me is the level of confidence I can now reach; the things I can do without alcohol. I was a confident teen but I wasn't a confident adult because I hid behind alcohol and used it to take me from level five to level eight, "socially confident". Now, I can dress in drag for a night out. I've gone from drinking half a litre of vodka a day to de-stress, to now enjoying life in the carefree way I did as a teenager. And I didn't even find it overly hard to quit.

Doctors should know better than to drink hard, but we tell ourselves we deserve it. We're saving lives, after all! It's arrogance, meets loneliness, meets self-destruction, meets entitlement.'

THE ANTI-JOY OF
UNEXPECTED TRIGGERS

There are triggers that are entirely expected. We know to anticipate the hand-twitch for beer sloshing out of a paper cup at a gig; the scratch for prosecco at a birthday bash; the awkward rictus-grin we'll find on our faces when our friends simultaneously slam a squadron of flamin' tequilas.

Gotcha. Duly warned. Thanx bye, Blatantly Obvious Committee.

However, there are many, many unexpected triggers that creep up behind us, ninja-like, tap us on the shoulder and kapow! us.

In early years, these unexpecteds come thick and fast. I know people who found the humdrum act of cooking dinner to be such a provocateur (*This is when you normally have me. I know you want me,* says the wine) that they had to subsist on takeaways and microwave meals for the first month.

I've heard of others who found that plane travel made them so trigger (un)happy – given their previous predilection for using 'airplane rules' to start drinking at 11am – that they had to get ferries or trains instead.

Still others that associated Europe (in particular France) with wine so much that they postponed travelling there until they felt steadier about sitting at a wobbly pavement table people-watching without wine.

Who knew that cooking, air travel and France could invoke alcohol cravings?!

Personally, one of the most triggery times in my first year was just before my soberversary. On day 364 sober. Don't ask me why. Something in me tripped. Said that given I'd been fucking things up for so long *before* these 364 days, that I was bound to fuck this up too, so I may as well have a drink already.

It was the 'Who do you think you are?' voice. The 'You have NOT got this!' voice, that whispered faster and faster as the date approached. And then, hallelujah, praise be, sing Hosanna! It shut the heck up.

But, there have been unexpected triggers that have appeared, and even intensified, in long-term recovery. So without further ado, here are my top four: summer, procrastination, PMT and illness.

Summer did some serious prodding of me in years five and six, while procrastination was always a special skill of mine, but in year seven (when lockdown hit), it stepped up a notch. PMT and illness are things I struggle with *even now*.

1. SUMMER

There's a trip switch flipped by one simple, inexorable change. The seasons.

For some, the problematic calendar gauntlet is that stretch between autumn and winter. They associate the temperature drop with supping mulled wine in front of a snap-crackle-pop fire. Or warming their frost-nibbled hands around a hot toddy. Or pushing their toes into a sheepskin rug, while red wine scorches the back of their throat.

But for me, it was all about summer's arrival. When the sky turned from dove-grey to kingfisher-blue. When the sun turned from a delicate disc to a ball o' fire, I experienced unexpected, urgent cravings.

It's not just me. There's something about sunshine that makes us want to sprint to a beer garden, inexplicably order rosé and throw it down our throats. 2017's British heatwave saw a £158 million surge in alcohol sales.

Why? Genius marketing. It's why we tend to jones for certain drinks at certain times. Warming whiskey in winter; Aperol spritz in summer. Irish cream when it's cold; ice-clinking cider when it's hot. If NASA did marketing campaigns, the machine around alcohol would be the result.

We're implicitly – or explicitly – told that getting drunk is the key to a sensational summer. Malibu uses the strapline 'Because Summer' in its campaigns. Martini depicts a red-dress-clad model dancing around Rome's cobbled streets. Orchard Thieves goes with sunshine-drenched rooftop parties. While the Bud Light ad features a beach shindig replete with Chinese lanterns, horse riding and dancing in animal masks around a bonfire (gimme an invite to that party).

Summer means jugs of Pimm's crowded with cucumber, mint and strawberries. But, it's just conditioning. We've become Pavlov's dogs, who salivated on the clang of the bell. Or Little Albert, the famous baby who played happily with a white rat, until he was conditioned into being scared of it. We're conditioned to crave booze in summer.

These smokescreens of marketing obscure the reality of what our summer drinking actually looked like. Has a white wine spritzer ever resulted in my going on a spontaneous trip to the coast in a convertible, to try on comedy sunglasses and jape around on an antique horse carousel? Nope.

Has one white wine spritzer led to six, and meant I've had to phone my boyfriend and slur 'come get me' after almost falling onto the train tracks at Wimbledon Station? Yup. Yes it has.

Because my sunshine drinking sessions always started so much earlier, they wound up being so much messier. 'Picnic on the common!' or 'rounders in the park' texts would stream about from 1pm on Saturday. In the summer, the opportunities to start drinking at lunchtime abounded.

And so, as the sun dipped, I gradually shed my belongings, dignity, romantic standards and ability to say three-syllable words successfully. Sunday would be spent wrapped in the duvet, self-loathing, with the dread of terse 'about last night' texts.

Whereas my sunny sober weekends feature 9am yoga, long river walks, exhibitions, comedy shows and feeling good all the damn time – not just for a couple of hours.

It's important, for me, to disentangle the seasonal-change marketing from the reality. I've summer-drank in search of those balmy convertible nights many, many times. And the definition of insanity is: doing the same thing over and over and expecting different results. Right? Right.

A happy hour or two is not worth the remainder of my weekend being unhappy. The beer garden is just as dappled, friendly and sparkly with elderflower pressé in my glass.

2. PROCRASTINATION

I frequently paired my wine with procrastination, back in the drinking day.

Hungover, I was a master procrastinator. I would spend an entire Friday fake-working at my desk, which consisted of bantering over email or stalking people I went to school with on Facebook. *Swoosh*: I would switch my screen to email or a Word document, should my boss walk past. When the clock chimed 5.31pm, I'd be outta the building like it was on fire. Ba-bye, chumps.

And then at 6am on Monday, I'd be punching the out-of-hours entry code into the door, sliding in shamefully, having stressed all weekend about *how much I had to do*, but drinking instead of *doing some of it*.

I would then bash at my computer, in the manner of *Sesame*

Street's Animal at the drums, wild-eyed and panting, until my co-workers came in, when I would be forced to act like a normal person. 'Who me?! I'm fine! Not an entire day behind.'

I soon learned in sobriety that I was going to need to temper this all-go or all-flop self-sabotage. My days were either pure procrastination or pure 'holy fucking shit' grind. I needed to find a speed between Frank *Shameless* and Sheryl Sandberg. And I did. Mostly achieved by using a co-working space.

Then lockdown landed in year seven and my co-working space was swiped away. Worst of all, I was placed in a room with my #1 procrastination enabler. My rectangular nemesis; the telly. I also use cleaning and exercise to procrastinate, but the TV is my ultimate adversary when it comes to getting shit done.

Turn me on, it whispered. *It's lunchtime*, it insisted. *Just one*, it coaxed.

I put a Post-it saying 'NO!' on the TV, to remind myself. And thxbutnothx to wireless headphones; I literally tether myself to my laptop using my ancient plug-in headphones, like you'd tie a dog to a chair. *Stay there.*

Thankfully, recovery teaches us that even though our brains might *want* something then and there, like three episodes of *Criminal Minds*, it's not a good idea. Just as a parent steers a toddler away from eating gravel or touching the pretty spikes.

3. PMT
If you'd asked me when I was drinking if I got Pre-Menstrual Tension (also known as PMS), I would have said 'nope'. Given I was usually hungover four or five times a week from 2008 to 2013, and the symptoms of a hangover are spookily similar to PMT, I had no clue that I suffered from it. I pretty much always felt on the verge of tears, like a lascivious hornball, or irrationally furious with the

world. That was me *all month long*.

If you're not aware, PMT feels like this. Your emotions are errant and random, pin-balling around inside you. Ding – anxiety. Ding – anger. Ding – horny. Ding – sadness. Where will the pinball go next? Nobody knows. One moment you want reassurance, then you want to rip someone's head off, then the lights dip and rhythm and grind plays – er, actually, how's about a shag?

So, it was almighty News To Me when I discovered that, as a sober, I experienced fierce PMT once a month, for at least three days. It's not an uncommon realisation. 'Say what? I get PMT? Who knew!' is a revelation I have seen hundreds of times online, in the sobersphere.

I'm PMT-ing (tension doesn't quite cover it; tyranny would be better) right now, in fact. I'm furious at the smoker I just walked behind, who I feel made me share their cigarette. At the strange man who stood too close while mansplaining something I already knew. At the app I'm trying to use for not working. At myself for getting into the office later than planned.

Reader, I am even angry at my hair today. My hair is being a right tosser.

Each and every month, I forget that this is about to happen, in some monthly fit of PMT amnesia, and when it does, it takes me a while to twig. Ahhhh, that's why I'm about as well-adjusted as Jack Nicholson in *The Shining*. That's why I keep having to re-listen to my 'Kind heart: cherishing others' Buddhist meditation like my life depends upon it!

It's clinically proven, of course. 'Anger and irritability are one of the most severe and persistent symptoms of PMS that adversely affect women,' said one clinical 2019 study (PMS is an umbrella term for all premenstrual symptoms, while PMT is used to telescope down to the 'tension' fall-out).

This study looked at 720 women and found that, 'the average scores of women with PMS for constant anger (anger-in and anger-out) was significantly higher' than those who weren't pre-menstrual. 'It is thought that hormonal changes in the menstrual cycle (fluctuations in estrogen and progesterone levels) affect the mood of women and trigger negative emotions such as anger and irritability,' the study adds.

What's more, we're 'more likely to seek out alcohol' during stages when our estrogen is high (it peaks just before our period lands), said a 2017 study.

'When estrogen levels are higher, alcohol is much more rewarding,' said the author of the study. Which makes you 'more likely to overindulge.' For all I know, my alcohol use was peaking just as my estrogen did, in order to muffle the PMT. I just didn't notice, because I was drunk.

As a sober, even though I intellectually know all of this anger is a biological fact, yet psychologically illogical, it doesn't remove how intense it feels. I can know that *I don't really hate* the smoker, the mansplainer, the app, myself or my tosser hair, but my body feels that way nonetheless. You can't think your way out of PMT.

I have no magical cure, no silver bullet that will slay this lunar-like cycle. Just like some British police forces report that the full moon coincides with people being more anti-social, all you can do is be aware of it. To know it's coming and – brace. Do nothing. Say nothing. React not.

And then, I get my period and the red mist lifts. Angels may as well start playing harps above me. Oh, happy day! The transformation is akin to Maleficent being turned into Mother Theresa. The horn removal is instant. It's just hormones; it's just science, and even though PMT can feel acutely like a spiritual bypass, it too shall pass. Just as the full moon waxes and wanes.

Happily, I also then begin to notice the flipside of the menstrual cycle. The whoosh! of energy and mood we tend to experience in week two of our cycle (generally just after our actual period has ended). Thanks to a spike in testosterone and estrogen, we can feel quicker, brighter, smarter, less prone to pain; basically like a newborn vampire without the unfortunate diet.

4. ILLNESS

As I write, I am quarantined at home with some lesser-spotted Covid-19 symptoms, during the crest of the second wave in the UK.

It's more than likely a cold. But, I was meant to be going to Cornwall tomorrow with my family. I realised last night that, given I smashed two Lemsips in a row (and Lemsip is rank), I probably shouldn't go.

The responsible-citizen thing to do is postpone it until I can be sure I'm not liable to kill off my vulnerable loved ones, and lock myself in my flat until I have a negative test result in my paw. Enter: solitary Covid-ment.

So, I've done the mature, responsible thing, right? I'm no super-spreader. I know that I'm definitely ill, because even standing up is challenging. And yet I feel anxious and guilty. Like a fraud, who has let her family down.

Why? Simple. There is a string in my head that *still*, even now, links feeling ill with being hungover. And so, feeling ill makes me feel hangdog guilty. The string goes: 'feels ill – cancels – bad person – guilt.'

It's no great surprise, really. During my 21 years of drinking, I was hangover-ill approximately 3,000 times. I was genuinely ill maybe 42 times. This means I was hangover-ill circa 71 times to every *one time* I was legitimately ill, so the connection is undeniably profound.

There's the physicality of it. My throat is scratchy, which reminds me of when I corroded my throat with cigarette smoke, dry ice and shouting over music so loud it made your teeth chatter.

My body needs to over-sleep, just as it did when hungover. I wake up after nine+ hours and instead of feeling glad my body has been regenerating, I feel clotted, thick with shame, given my body and mind link the over-sleep so strongly with the drinking.

There's the necessity of resting. It's now entirely legitimate, crucial even, for me to lie down and watch kids' films like *Abominable**, read books, eat steaming ramen and nap, but doing so gives me the skin-pricking feeling that I'm doing something wrong.

My logical brain knows that there's nothing to feel anxious or guilty about, yet this episode has plucked some subterranean part of my lizard brain, which is now telling me, 'Did you get smashed in Soho again? Wine-flu, *again*? You bad dipsomaniac! I can't believe you're letting your family down *again*. You're going to hell. Give our regards to Attila the Hun, you'll probably share a bunk with him, Cath.'

It makes absolutely no sense, but it's there.

My muscle memory doesn't believe in my illness, even when it's irrefutably true. I'll be told by a pharmacist: 'You need to go home and rest.' And as I'm texting my loved ones to cancel our Sunday lunch date – even though I am telling the God's Honest – I feel like I'm lying, because the composing of that text tweaks the visceral part of me that says: *when I cancel, I'm lying.* Even when I'm not lying.

---

* I just had this conversation with a Bulgarian friend. Me: 'I'm gonna watch *Abominable*.' Him: 'A bum and a bull?' Me: 'Yes, abominable.' Him: 'Like, a bum and also a bull?' Once we'd untangled the lost-in-translation misunderstanding, we spiralled off into planning a storybook series, given kids find bums and bulls hilarious. In the series, we'll also release 'A fart and a fox' and 'A wee and a wallaby'. Crowdfunder: pending.

A GP will have confirmed that a stomach parasite has hitched a ride with me from Thailand, which is why I look five months pregnant and constantly feel nauseous, but I will feel like a charlatan when I cancel a work commitment.

Being ill makes me feel lost, even now. Like I've been plunged back into the darkness. And so I have to parent the shit out of myself when I'm ill. I have to write myself reassuring 'Everything is OK' lists where I tell myself that I'm not a bad person, just an ill one.

'Are we back there?', says a very small voice inside me. And I have to pull it onto my lap, and stroke its hair back from its forehead, kiss it and say – *no, my sweet, we are not. You just rest. Get better.*

READERS ON THEIR UNEXPECTED TRIGGERS

'Big-event sex. Role play, BDSM and sex parties were always attended while buzzed. Even now, being sober during creative or non-vanilla sex feels a bit... wrong? It doesn't actually change anything; you still get into it, but the initial awkwardness makes me crave shots like nothing else.'

Ava

'Losing or misplacing something. It reminds me of my drunk, haphazard ways, when I would leave half of my life scattered around London.'

Kate

'Having had an amazingly productive day. It triggers that feeling of, "I've achieved lots, so I deserve wine!" when, in fact, the lack of alcohol is the reason I was productive.'

Violet

'Mine was, paradoxically, the ordinary. We know about the big-picture stuff – new job, moving house – and put self-care mechanisms in. So I was blindsided by the day-to-day, like long Sunday walks ending in the pub. These were my potential banana skins for which I had to be vigilant; not just the big-ticket items.'

Hazel

'I love fashion. I drank at home pretty often while organising, sorting and trying things on in my closet. Pre-picking outfits for work and leisure. When I stopped drinking, it felt like something was missing during my closet rotation, so I actually had to take a break from self-styling sessions. But I refused to let it stick. Now I style sober. Wine cannot take the credit for my style creativity any more!'

Portia

'When I see a fictional character on TV drinking alcohol. Them enjoying themselves at a party? Wine. Consoling themselves after some bad news? Wine. Somehow seeing it on screen does something in my brain that tells me to pour a glass of wine, almost as if I'm in the company of the people on TV. Weird.'

Taylor

'Making phone calls to family, especially my mom. My sobriety is mostly straightforward and craving-free, but I continue to struggle with this! I now make sparkling-water concoctions while on the phone, to ease it.'

Jameela

'I stopped drinking because I thought it was making my marriage hard. When I stopped, I realised that it was my marriage being hard that had triggered me. I thought it was chicken then egg, but really it was egg then chicken.'

Dee

STONE COLD VS SUNSHINE WARM ANGER

STONE COLD DRUNK ANGER

DECEMBER 2010

If I'm angry with someone, I feel entitled to tell them. To punish them. The very presence of my anger is evidence that I am Right and they are Wrong. If I feel it, it must be righteous, and so I must unleash it in order to burn the injustice to embers.

If a friend suggests that maybe I don't come to her birthday, given I've had big fall-outs with three of the attendees, I send her an email saying how 'outrageous' her suggestion is, and 'How dare you put them above me?'.

If a stranger is 'rude' to me, I don't contemplate the novel notion that perhaps I misunderstood, or they're just having a fucker of a day; I take it intensely personally. I glare at them, my eyeballs boring holes in the back of their head. I even 'squash their head' Fonejacker-style, with my thumb and forefinger, when they're far enough away.

My anger is a fire-breathing pet dragon that I feed, stroke and tend to, before sending it out into the world to wreak vengeance and desolation. I don't see my anger as mine to hold; an irrational knee-jerk, or an entirely human but often illogical emotion.

I am wrong.

SUNSHINE WARM SOBER ANGER

I no longer send my anger out into the world in the shape of poison-pen emails, venomous text messages or actual handwritten letters (so Nineties!). I now understand that my anger is my responsibility; not necessarily an accurate barometer. And it's most certainly not a bat I'm entitled to bash people with.

In the first few years of sobriety, the very presence of anger fizzing in my system made me feel like A Bad Person. 'Anger is a luxury we cannot afford,' I heard recited often, in the sobersphere. As if anger is caviar, cashmere or Fabergé eggs.

On the contrary, I think anger is an essential we have to *afford. Denying the existence of anger is dangerous. Locked inside, anger can become an imploding star, which creates a black hole.*

And so I did a lot of work around reconciling the fact I am allowed to feel the full spectrum of emotions. I am allowed to feel the rainbow, as are you; even the storm-violet of anger. I forgive myself for the anger. I weather it. And I move through it. Into the buttercup-yellow.

The healthiest sober people I know allow themselves to feel anger, to process it, without inflicting it upon others. They're the ones who go into the middle of nowhere and indulge in a bit of forest-screaming, followed by some forest-bathing. They're the ones who vent it in safe rooms (therapy, meetings, their aunt's conservatory), rather than feign beatific never-anger.

The mark of A Good Person is not never feeling anger; it's what we do with that anger. Whether we allow it to escape and flame-tongue our loved ones, burning our personal worlds to the ground. Or if we name it, leash it, train it, exercise it and soothe it in privacy instead. Anger isn't bad, per se. *It just is.*

It really helped me when I read First, We Make the Beast Beautiful *by Sarah Wilson, and she relayed that the Dalai Lama runs his anger away on a treadmill. I delighted in the mental image of His Holiness pounding a treadmill, ideally wearing his scarlet-and-gold robes, with anger lava running through his veins. It was a comfort. Him turning his smoulder into a glow, through the chemistry conversion of cortisol expulsion and endorphin creation.*

I think of the Dalai Lama on that treadmill often.

NEW CELEBRITY ENTRIES TO SOBER VILLAGE

There's no greater leveller than addiction. It doesn't matter if you have a swimming pool and a chauffeur, you're not immune. Addiction doesn't care if you have an Oscar, or have been voted the world's sexiest rapper. Swag can't buy you sobriety.

Finding out that some star you've never met is also sober draws a star-hung line of connection from your humble gaffe in Manchester to their chi-chi crib in Manhattan. *Elton John's sober too?! ELTON, my buddy!*

You feel like you know them all of a sudden. Even though you don't. And yet, you do know the same feeling, intimately. The Ultimate Shared Experience of staring into the abyss, and the abyss staring back, and you deciding, 'Y'know what? No ta.'

I'll often watch films and hug the knowledge that Robert Downey Jr, or Jada Pinkett Smith, or Tom Hardy, or Kerry Washington are sober too. In the early days, the knowledge that they were sober and killing it kept me going.

I also loved knowing that even if they played big-drinkin' characters, they were sober behind-the-scenes. Colin Farrell plays a beer 'n' chaser fiend in *True Detective*, but is many years sober in real life. Actual Christina Ricci drinks Diet Coke in nightclubs, but celluloid Christina glides around with martinis while playing Zelda Fitzgerald. Gillian Jacobs, star of *Love*, appears in films wearing sweatshirts saying things like 'Alcohol you later', but has never had a drink in her entire life.

Some may see sober celebrity lists as shallow, and to those people I say – *it's only a bit of fun*. Go frown into some Kafka and leave us be.

Ready for some sober celebrity star-gazing? Let's go.

KATE MOSS

She's always been the silent, enigmatic snow leopard of celebrities, whose motto is, 'Never complain, never explain', so Kate hasn't talked about sobriety herself, but those close to her have.

Her sister Lottie told the *Daily Mail* in 2018 that, 'Kate is not drinking any more, she is fully clean.'

This was then backed up by her close buddy, DJ Fat Tony (also sober himself) in June 2020, who revealed, 'Kate's been clean for over two years. Me and my sober mates now have a better time than we ever did when we used to drink and take drugs.'

THUNDERCAT

His breakthrough album was *Drunk*, featuring many lyrics that explored addiction, such as in the title track 'Drunk', ('Drowning away all of the pain/ 'til I'm totally numb') or 'Drink Dat' ('Pourin' shots, ain't worried 'bout precautions or the cost'/ 'Cause we goin' far, another drink, it might be a problem'/ 'I can't...'/ 'Can't open my eyes, girl') and yet Thundercat is always sober as a ~~judge~~ juggernaut on stage.

'I took some time to revamp and look at myself and turn things into something else. I stopped drinking,' he told *Vulture*. 'Immediately, I lost a lot of weight. It was kind of scary for people who were friends of mine, because they thought I was on drugs or something. It was a bit anxious for me at first, with everything between withdrawal and emotions. It was a lot to take on. Everything would be coming at me pretty fast. But I got used to it. I found my rhythm in it.'

JESSICA SIMPSON

She hasn't had a drink since 2017. 'Giving up the alcohol was easy,' she writes in her memoir, *Open Book*. 'I was mad at that bottle. At how it allowed me to stay complacent and numb.' She added on Sirius XM: 'I thought it was making me brave, I thought it was making me confident and it was actually the complete opposite.'

STEPHEN KING

'The hungover eye,' he once wrote in a novel, 'had a weird ability to find the ugliest things in any given landscape.' Turns out King writes car-crash rock bottoms *really well* because he's been sober himself since the late Eighties. But his own bottom was nowhere near as theatrical as his characters'. 'I don't have anything as dramatic,' Stephen told the *Guardian*. 'Of course, in a novel, you're looking for something that's really harsh. Harshly lit. For me, when I look back, the thing that I remember is being at one of my son's Little League games with a can of beer in a paper bag, and the coach coming over to me and saying, "If that's an alcoholic beverage, you're going to have to leave".'

MEG MATHEWS

'I was in my early 40s when I realised that partying wasn't for me any more and I had to get myself into a better situation,' Meg Mathews told the *Sun*, about her quit in 2016. 'You can't go on living like that for ever, staying up all night, not eating properly, drinking...I don't have alcohol in the house and I don't give it a thought. I can't just have one or two glasses of wine... going for "a couple of drinks" isn't in my vocabulary, so I might as well forget that. I'm all or nothing, that's me. So I think it's better that I just don't have any. I don't want to wake up feeling groggy. I want to wake up feeling clear.'

KENDRICK LAMAR

Now an advocate for clean-living, sober Lamar alluded to his former drinking as a fitting-in attempt in the song 'Swimming Pools': 'Some people like the way it feels/ Some people wanna kill their sorrows/ Some people wanna fit in with the popular, that was my problem.'

LILY ALLEN

Lily celebrated her first year sober in July 2020. Talking to *GQ* magazine, she said, 'I was drinking a bottle of Grey Goose a day. It was really bad.'

One memorable convincer involved head-butting herself unconscious while on Orlando Bloom's lap, which triggered an intervention by Chris Martin (reportedly also sober himself).

'I was very, very drunk and I head-butted something behind Orlando Bloom and knocked myself out,' she explained to *E! News*. 'Then Chris Martin, who is a friend of mine, and Gwyneth, who is a close friend of my mom, drove me home. He [Chris] left a Post-it note on my fridge just saying, "Give me a call tomorrow". I did.'

ANTHONY HOPKINS

Talking about being 45 years sober in *Interview* magazine, Anthony said, 'I look at it, and I think, "What a great blessing that was, because it was painful." I did some bad things. But it was all for a reason, in a way. And it's strange to look back and think, "God, I did all those things?" But it's like there's an inner voice that says, "It's over. Done. Move on".'

LEONA LEWIS

She hasn't drunk in years, says it tastes 'like hairspray', and has a great time without alcohol. Talking to *Fabulous* magazine, Leona referenced Amy Winehouse, who tragically died from alcohol poisoning aged 27, saying, 'It would probably have been very easy for me to have been like Amy.'

JOHN MAYER

His quit was inspired by a gargantuan six-day hangover after Drake's 30th birthday party. 'That's how big the hangover was,' he said. 'I looked out the window and I went, "OK, John, what percentage of your potential would you like to have? Because if you say you'd like 60, and you'd like to spend the other 40 having fun, that's fine. But what percentage of what is available to you would you like to make happen? There's no wrong answer. What is it?" I went, "100."

John wishes there was more 'sober-enabling' on social media. 'You have to fight really hard to look at it from a critical point of view because it's constantly pushed on you. Every Friday and Saturday on social media there is enabling that is going on for drinking. What if I woke up every morning on Saturday and Sunday and put my feet on the ground and I just went, "Not hungover!" And put it on social media every day. You forget that's an option.' Hear, hear, John.

PEARL LOWE

'I've been sober nearly 15 years now,' she said on *Loose Women*. 'When I look at old pictures I just think, "My God, who is that person?" I actually look at pictures and think "I feel quite sorry for her" because I was in pain and it seemed like it was this great place to be, at all these parties, but I had young children and I was trying to keep my husband happy, be happy, go out and try to have a career – because I was in a band at the time – but it was so difficult and obviously something had to give. Basically, I ended up getting rid of my mobile phone and moving to the country.'

50 CENT

The rapper doesn't drink 'in da club', even when it looks like he is. He invests heavily in a line of champagne, so to market it, he performs a sleight of hand on the 'bottle full of bub'.

'First I'll pour drinks from a bottle of champagne for everyone who is in VIP with me. When the bottle is empty, I'll give it to one of my guys and have him quietly refill it with ginger ale,' he writes in his memoir, *Hustle Harder, Hustle Smarter*. 'For the rest of the night I'll have that bottle in my hand. I'll take swigs every now and then just to keep the vibe right, but I'm not drinking anything but Canada Dry.'

LENA DUNHAM

'Being sober in life is hard,' Lena Dunham told *Variety*. 'But being sober is the first step to facing all the things that made you want to hide in the first place.'

Lena's admitted on *The Jonathan Ross Show* that she's found sober dating, particularly in the UK, challenging: 'Sober dating in the UK is a roughie. It was easy to find guys when I would drink because I would drink a lot, go over to their house, throw up and then they would have to let me stay. But in Wales when I was being a polite woman of dignity and grace? Much more challenging.'

Speaking at a benefit luncheon for a women-only rehab, Lena also said: 'Being me has sometimes hurt so much that I couldn't bear it. But being me is also a super-power, and it's the same for all of you. And I'll put my money on sober women any day – because a woman who has overcome an addiction can do f–ing anything.'

DAVID SEDARIS

The straight-up hilarious essayist and novelist is now teetotal. 'I had been wanting to quit for a long time. I was afraid to quit, afraid that

I wouldn't be able to write, because I started drinking shortly after I started writing,' says David. 'And then I kind of got it in my head that I needed to be drinking while I wrote. ...I don't know why I was so convinced of it, it's like saying "I can't sing unless I have a blue shirt on".

JAMEELA JAMIL

Jameela has never drunk alcohol and is bewildered by the societal pushback she gets. 'Most people when I tell them this, look at me as though I've just told them, very casually, that I like to eat people,' Jameela says. 'It's always met with suspicion and a demand to know my reasoning. I just decided very young that I didn't want to trick myself into thinking I'm having a good time when I'm not. I didn't want to lose my vulnerability when I felt shy or afraid. I didn't want to lose my wits about me, especially as a young woman. And I didn't like the look of hangovers, what it does to people's looks and mostly what it does to people's bank accounts. The cons didn't seem worth the pros to me.'

BRAD PITT

Not actually a new entry, but he said something recently that captured something I believe fiercely in: the focus on 'what the person does next'. So, I made an exception. You're welcome, Brad ;-)

'We've always placed great importance on the mistake,' Brad said in *Interview* magazine, referencing addicted drinking. 'But the next move, what you do after the mistake, is what really defines a person. We're all going to make mistakes. But what is that next step? We don't, as a culture, seem to stick around to see what that person's next step is. And that's the part I find so much more invigorating and interesting.'

Wild applause to that, Brad. What comes next is what defines us.

BURNING QUESTION: ONCE AN ADDICT, ALWAYS AN ADDICT?

Dr Marc Lewis says: 'People quit all the time. The stats are clear. More than half of those with a substance-use disorder stop – and more than half of those quit without any sort of formal treatment.

For some people, the "once an addict, always an addict" narrative is a real cross to bear. It increases pessimism and reduces the sense of being an evolving, transforming person. You feel stuck in a certain pattern for ever.'

Dr Judith Grisel says: 'To me as a recovering addict, if we're talking in terms of drinking or using again, testing that theory out would be like trying to test out if I can fly. Which involves jumping off that roof. It feels like a bad bet to me! There's no good evidence that shows you can go back to moderate use after having been addicted.'

Dr David Nutt says: 'Well, the vulnerability for addiction – whether genetic or acquired – never goes away. And you're always going to be more vulnerable to addiction once you've succumbed to it. Your brain learns addiction just as it learns to ride a bike, so your brain will remember.

There's a strange biological phenomenon in that it can take you four or five years to learn an addiction, say, but then even after many years of abstinence, your usage can shoot back up to what it was previously within a few weeks of re-using. The vulnerability to addiction will always be there, even when the craving is not.'

Dr Julia Lewis says: 'Humans are messed-up bundles of extremely complicated carbon, so we don't know this for sure, but studies suggest that after four to five years of solid abstinence, you're considered "stable" in recovery. That doesn't mean you should go out and drink or use again, but it's also true that your brain won't be a slave to that former addiction forevermore. The brain is very plastic. Adaptable. The part that previously lit up and nudged you to drink can be repurposed to light up and trigger you to exercise, or something else that's good for you.'

NOTES ON THE 'JUST AN ADDICT' NARRATIVE

I recently sat watching a six-years-sober friend literally pour sour candy into his open mouth, as one might pour water from a jug into a glass. 'I can't stop, Cath. I'm just an addict.' I laughed, but it troubled me. A week later, I sipped tea with another friend, also a long-time sober, who told me that he couldn't stop using porn, because he's 'just an addict'.

The 'just an addict' narrative is like an albatross many of us wear around our necks for eternity. It makes me profoundly sad when I hear sober warriors, who have five, ten, fifteen years sober, say things like, 'I can't quit smoking/overeating/drinking coffee because, after all, I'm *just an addict*.' Whether 'just an addict' is said in a world-weary resigned tone, or in a cheerful gallows tone, I flinch every dang time.

If you have overcome an addiction, you're not *just an addict*. I want to hoist you onto my shoulders and do a lap of glory with you. You've had the grit and grace to take a long hard look at yourself, to excavate all the things – both the dirty and the pretty – and take inventory of them, deciding what to keep and what to (try to) discard. Not many people on this planet have the wisdom and courage to do that.

You're not JUST an addict. You're someone who has traversed that battlefield and emerged victorious. Yes, you may add the disclaimer 'won *for now*', if that's your preference. But whether 'for now' or 'for ever', you've still done that! Nobody can take that time away from you, whether it's one year or 50. You're someone who has stared down an addiction and won. If I ever go into a fray with addiction, I want you by my side, not some charmed-life poppet.

Yes, when people quit an all-consuming primary addiction, such as daily drinking, they tend to grab a secondary addiction to plug that super-massive black hole. That's true. But it doesn't mean they are predestined to do battle with ever-coming addictions for the rest of their days. There is no proof for that; any reportage of it is purely anecdotal.

Those who have now beaten a primary addiction are tooled-up, battle-stripe-wearing and shark-tooth-carrying* survivors. You are *more* able to whack that secondary, third, fourth addiction that pops its mole head up than your common-or-garden human. Just because you were addicted to some stuff in the past, it doesn't mean you are a special subsect of human who shall continue to get addicted to everything.

As for those who are merely here on some sober-curious tourism to see if they fancy living here, you are courageous too. Most people ostrich-head, living their entire lives without looking hard at themselves + the thing in their hand. The process of quitting drinking, whether 'for now' or for ever, starts long before the last drink. You're already in the process, merely by reading this book.

Addiction is a universal experience

Becoming addicted to something, at some point in our lives, is an utterly universal human experience. I can't think of one person, not one, who isn't addicted to *something*. Can you, honestly, when you really think about it?

There's my friend who doesn't have Wi-Fi, because he'll end

---

* Metaphorical. Please only actually wear a shark's tooth if you would be OK with a shark wearing human teeth as earrings.

up watching Netflix 'til 4am. There's my friend who tried to quit Diet Coke, announcing 'I've quit!' publicly for accountability, and found herself sneaking it in the toilets at work. There's the co-worker who's addicted to hitting 'refresh' on the news and thriving on the breathless hyperbole of passing the doom on to others. There's my friend who can't sit down for an hour's lunch with me without checking her text messages five times and even tapping out responses.

Speaking of which, phones are our new addictive nemesis. I was lucky enough to go on a spa weekend recently, and beside the pool, at least three-quarters of loungers were staring at their phones. In the jacuzzi? About half, taking selfies. They filmed each other doing the ice bucket, doing the polar-bear plunge, diving into the pool. Then watched the replays, rather than enjoy the actual experience. If these people could have taken their phones into the sauna, they would've.

None of these people have officially worn the 'addict' label, either voluntarily or involuntarily. But they do have addictions. They're just undiagnosed by society, or themselves, because their addictions are less visible and don't involve public humiliation where you slur, stagger and break furnishings.

Some of these addictions are even actively encouraged by corners of society (phone, work, social media, news, shopping; I could go on). The darkest places these socially accepted addictions may take these people may be to a bathroom stall, where they chug Diet Coke, but that doesn't make it any less of an addiction.

Why our stories are self-fulfilling prophecies

Our lived experience tends to follow what we think is going to happen. It's confirmation bias supersized, but instead of seeing what we expect to, we live out what we expect to. Maybe you do keep getting addicted to things – sugar, exercise, coffee – now you've quit drinking.

But did your experience follow your opinions? Or did you shape your story with your expectations? Did you pour it into a jelly mould and then go, 'Goshdarnit, whaddayaknow! This jelly is shaped like a rabbit!' Course it is. You poured it in there, buddy. This is why we need to choose what stories we pour our sobriety into very carefully.

If you see yourself as a hopelessly devoted, who shall now spend the rest of their days craving a long-lost paramour, your sobriety will feel like that. The power of the stories you believe, and then re-tell yourself, is profound in the extreme. It's a coat hanger you hang the rest of your life upon.

Noting the GPS of the cliff edge

'It only takes one day, one slip, to re-set it all to zero,' someone in long-term recovery said to me recently. My eyes pricked with tears and I felt an overwhelming urge to hug him, despite that being practically illegal in pandemic Britain. 'If you've done five years, you're more than capable of for ever,' I said, softly. But he stared back at me from his cliff edge and shook his head.

This 'cliff-edge mentality' is the ultimate psychological catch-22. Many in recovery believe that unless us recoverees eyeball the cliff edge we could somersault over at any time, then peril beckons. We'll accidentally tumble over it. 'Watch the edge!' this mentality urges.

Of course, the edge exists. It would be foolish to pretend it doesn't. But to me, staring at it constantly would be like an open-heart surgeon consistently reminding themselves they could kill a patient at any second, or a tight-rope walker staring down instead of keeping their gaze level.

You don't have to gawk at the cliff edge daily, hourly, in order to avoid going arse over tit into an abyss filled with cider. We can just live somewhere else, note the GPS location of the edge, flag when we're coming close to it and resolve to stay away.

As 'cliff-edge man' and I stared at each other that day, something became clear to me. Where I live (far from the cliff edge) unsettles him. Where he lives (on the cliff edge) unsettles me. Neither of us is right, or wrong, we just *are*. But I know where I prefer to live.

WHAT IT'S LIKE TO BE THE ONLY ONE IN THE ROOM

The sober space is alarmingly – like many spaces – white. We need to change this. Addiction in BIPOC communities is not, as far as I've seen, any lower, so why is the visible sober community not reflecting the actual diversity ratio of those struggling and/or recovering?

I've been a fan of Laura Cathcart Robbins's brilliant work for a while now. She's the host of *The Only One in the Room* podcast. Clue's in the name. And given I have never been the only white person in any room, ever (even in recovery meetings in the Philippines), I asked Laura to write an essay for us.

She imparts some very important wisdom that we should all heed, particularly regarding the BIPOC community being silenced in meetings, when they discuss racism. I have never heard *anyone* be told that domestic violence, childhood trauma, divorce, so on and so forth are an 'outside issue' in a meeting, so why is racism? Anything that is a drinking trigger is an 'inside issue', frankly.

Over to Laura.

Why do all the Black people sit together in recovery meetings?

By Laura Cathcart Robbins

It's taken ten years.

Ten years of showing up at this women's meeting every Monday night. Ten years of asking other Black women to meet me here and then praying that all these well-intentioned white women are on their best behaviour. Not loudly marvelling at their hair ('How do you get it like that?') or putting them off with micro-aggressions, like 'What are you mixed with?' or 'Wow! You're so articulate!'

It took ten years to assemble a small group of Black women who feel safe enough to share freely in this nearly-all-white space. Each time a Black newcomer walks in the door, it's like one of us has arrived via the Underground Railroad, and our little band of 'others' is there to welcome her. We are a small brown oasis in a sea of white faces.

It's OK, sister girl, we see you. Come sit with us.

For me, this began when I was a kid, and I started flying round-trip from my mother's home in Cambridge, Massachusetts, to Fort Myers, Florida, to see my father. There weren't any cell phones back then, so my parents had no way to connect with me until I reached the arrival gate. This meant that they were obligated to rely on the white flight attendants' professionalism and kindness to whose care I was entrusted (I don't remember seeing a Black flight attendant until I was at least 13).

I can only imagine how terrifying it must have been for two African-Americans who'd grown up during Jim Crow to put their only child on a plane surrounded solely by white people. And to start doing so only seven short years after Lyndon B. Johnson signed the Civil Rights Act into law. Each time I boarded a flight, my father would look me in the eyes and solemnly offer me the same piece of advice:

'Remember, if you're lost, or you're in trouble, always look for a sister.'

Not a nun, mind you; we were never a religious family. No, my father was inferring that if I felt unsafe, she, whoever this woman was, would be a person that I could trust to help me. And so, at age six, I began a life-long habit of surveying any space that I might enter for an ally like the one my father spoke of – a Black woman.

In 2008, at 43 years old, I left an all-white Arizona treatment centre and entered the world of nearly all-white recovery meetings in Los Angeles.

It was a bumpy ride.

I was mid-divorce with two young boys. I was defiant, humiliated and shamed, and loath to admit that I was an alcoholic. And when I walked into the first meeting in LA, I paused in the doorway and surveyed the room. I was looking for a sister but found that I was the only one there darker than a paper bag.

The longer I stood there, the more attention I seemed to attract. I felt myself turning crimson as all of those white faces turned toward me to smile and inspect me as though I were the toy in a cereal box – like I was a prize. I took my seat, but I kept my head down, still feeling very much in the spotlight. I had no one to turn to, no one to give me 'the nod of recognition', no one to help buffer the sting of feeling like the only one in the room.

After a few months, I stopped focusing on the differences and managed to find some similarities. The woman in the seat next to mine was another newly divorced, the blonde sharing from the podium was a pill head like me, and that woman with the dope glasses spoke about the shame of being a drunk mom. You see, the rub was I wanted to be sober more than anything, and I understood in my core that these meetings were saving my life. But as months went by, I became even more aware of another thing that I needed – affinity. I was surprised by how great the need was for me to be witnessed by other Black people in recovery.

Fast forward 11 years, and there's been another layer to my struggle. The police are murdering American Black men and women in droves. And every time they take a Black life, I head to a meeting. But when I and others bring up racism in recovery meetings, we risk being admonished and informed that race is an outside issue.

Over the years, this has led to a PTSD-type response for me whenever race and recovery intersect. There was a long period where the other Black women and I did not feel safe discussing race in our homegroup. And as a result, these sisters and I stopped attending the meeting altogether, choosing BIPOC and POC recovery meetings instead.

Over the summer, several (white) women in my homegroup reached out to me to let me know that our absence was very much felt and our presence was missed. And while I appreciated the effort to connect, it was weeks before I was ready to reciprocate the sentiment. But this week, I feel as though something has shifted. I think I might want to drop in on my homegroup – the meeting that saved my life 12 years ago.

What about the next Black woman that Zooms or walks into my homegroup meeting and finds that she is the only one in the room? Will she leave because she feels alone, or will she be desperate enough to stay? If our primary purpose is to stay sober and carry the message, how can I do that if I'm not there?

One of my favourite women, a sister, walked into that same meeting five years ago and told me that she stayed solely because there was another Black woman there. Next Monday night, I think I'll join my homegroup for the first time in seven months.

And if another sister pops in to check out the meeting, I hope that she stays.

***

Laura Cathcart Robbins is a freelance culture writer and host of the popular podcast, *The Only One in The Room*, living in Studio City, California. Her recent articles in *HuffPo* and *The Temper* on the subjects of race, recovery and divorce have garnered her worldwide acclaim. Find out more about her at www.theonlyonepod.com, or you can look for her on Instagram @lauracathcartrobbins.

FURTHER READING TO TICKLE YOUR SOBER PICKLE

As we've just experienced, words are transportive. They can enable you to appreciate another's POV in the most profound, existential way. They can facilitate a tectonic shift of the mind. And they can also remind you of that which you've experienced – but have now clean forgotten. *Why am I not in a bar right now?! I loved drinking!* Er, no you didn't. That's why you quit, 'member?

Whenever I feel my thoughts sliding back towards bathing drinking in a rosy glow, or oblivion crooking its finger and telling me to 'come hither, my pretty', I always, always pick up a book.

Drinking romanticisation is like an insect bite. It niggles, demanding you attend to it. If you do scratch it, by ruminating on *all the things you miss about drinking* (really?), and forgetting all the reasons you quit, that poison will sure-as-hell spread. It will become mad, bad and dangerous to know.

Sitting with the itch, ignoring it, trusting it will go away, is only for the most advanced among us. See: those who can meditate for a half hour, despite a dripping tap. For us mere humans (*waggles hand* ME!), what I suggest is: a lightning bolt of knowledge.

I once grew very popular on a Mexican holiday for having something we named 'the clicker'. This tiny device went 'click' (shocker, I know) and gave an insect bite an infinitesimal electric shock. You could even *see* the miniature lightning bolt, which was extremely satisfying. It didn't actually scratch the itch, but it felt like it did. And so it provided relief while the tiny mosquito entry wound healed.

Learning about addiction, reading memoirs and geeking out

on neuroscience, is the equivalent of 'the clicker'. It's a jolt of relief. An 'ahhh, that feels better'. We blaze new thought-trails in our brains by reading books that disrupt the 'drinking good, sober bad' narrative. A narrative that is hurled at us hundreds of times a day in subliminal ways.

And so, without further ado, here are my favourite additions to the addiction canon, over the past few years.

QUIT LIKE A WOMAN BY HOLLY WHITAKER

Just as Kamala Harris (with an arched eyebrow – minx) praised Joe Biden for having 'the audacity' to choose a woman as a running mate, I applaud Holly for having 'the audacity' to write this book.

It placed her in the firing line for criticism, trolling and droves of lost followers. But she did it anyway. Because – fuck it. And that takes serious grit.

Holly has long been one of my favourite writers. Her sentence construction is often curveball intriguing, with a punchline of whipcrack wit that you rarely see coming.

At times righteous and unflinching, at others tender and vulnerable, Holly bravely dismantles the American recovery machine despite the risk of it blowing up in her face: rehab, AA, the disease model and so on. She takes a chainsaw to the status quo and our received wisdoms. And then painstakingly rebuilds.

The research she has done is vast, especially when drawing masterful parallels between Big Tobacco way-back-when and Big Alcohol now. Did you know that Big Tobacco once peddled the 'moderation is entirely possible and the norm' narrative? The one that is central to Big Alcohol's playbook? Yup. I didn't either, until Holly somehow excavated quotes from 1920s physicians.

Politicising aside, there's a really helpful and meticulously researched mid-section on our finite reserves of willpower, habit formation and dispatching cravings.

There are times when her arguments verge on radicalised. For instance, I agree that alcohol has been marketed to women as a badge of feminist rebellion (Johnnie Walker whiskey released 'Jane Walker' to celebrate women's rights – ugh), but I think it's a stretch to say that the motive for this is feminist subjugation ('a substance that is marketed to you to keep you from your power'). I think it's probably the simple vulgarity of profit margins.

But that's OK. I don't always have to agree with Holly in order to sit, rapt, as she tells personal stories laced with shivs of razorblade humour, and she soapboxes about personal recovery being a miniaturised revolution.

Best for: Womxn, frankly. Clue's in the title.

Not for: The most devoted of AAers, unless they're especially zen about hearing alternative viewpoints.

DRINK? BY PROFESSOR DAVID NUTT

This book turned me into a split-personality reader. I found myself punching the air, going 'Yes, David!' at some points, and scribbling angrily 'No, David!' in the column at others.

Why? He's wearing two hats throughout. First up is his 'work hat'. He was the government's chief drug adviser for many years and has spent his working life pointing out the roughshod wake of alcohol. But the second is a 'personal hat'; he's the co-owner of a wine bar who likes drinking, apparently finds moderation easy, thinks moderation is the ideal, and forgets that most of his readers are probably already sober, or aiming to be sober.

These two hats lead to contradictory zigzags. Allow me to demonstrate.

Zig: 'The drinks industry knows alcohol is a toxic substance. If it were discovered today, it would be illegal as a foodstuff. The safe limit of alcohol, if you applied food-standards criteria, would be one glass of wine a year.' (*David drops mic*).

Zag: 'Alcohol is such a powerful enabler of sociability and good humour; vital needs for most humans.' (And yet sociability, warmth and good humour are all entirely accessible without alcohol!)

Nonetheless, the zigs are worth the zags, because this is an absolute goldmine of data, research and trivia (in Japan, it's considered outrageously rude to leave a bar before your boss, hence the proliferation of 'tiny hotels' in business districts for people to crawl into at 3am).

Given he's so pro-alcohol (in moderation, mind) when wearing his personal hat, it makes it all the more profound and powerful when he rails against the corruption between the government and Big Alcohol. He's had a front-row seat to much of the muffling of alcohol harm, which makes for an ultra-fascinating section.

Best for: Eye-opening, sometimes startling analysis of alcohol studies.

Not for: Those who find the chatting up of moderation to be a trigger.

WE ARE THE LUCKIEST BY LAURA MCKOWEN

Laura writes with fiction-level poetic detail. Her style – in which sounds, smells and precise emotions are recalled flawlessly – reminds me of Lisa Taddeo (who wrote *Three Women*). Reading this, I felt her despair and euphoria as keenly as I feel my own emotions. That is a skill few writers have. Laura has it.

With courage, she explores her past drink-driving, drink-parenting and drink-cheating. A generous and welcome salve for those of us who have, at some point, done the same (read: thousands of us).

She writes beautifully about the shape-shifting many of us do to 'earn' love; the way we contort to avoid criticism and judgement, as if it were deadly, and switching from the dozen versions of ourselves (drinking) into the satisfyingly unfractured *one version* (sober).

Best for: A lose-yourself duvet day. This is a balm for parents who still feel guilt for drinking around their children.

Not for: Given it's a straight-up memoir, it swivels to take in the outside world very little, so if you're looking for stats, experts or a cultural sweep, look elsewhere.

THE SOBER LUSH BY AMANDA EYRE WARD AND JARDINE LIBAIRE

This gorgeous book pays homage to the notion that ex-drinkers are still hedonists who need their kicks; just not kicks served in margarita glasses rimmed with salt.

Insightful observations about sobriety arc sprinkled through what is essentially an anthology of ideas of what to do with your newfound sober life. Like the adrenaline spike of a polar-bear plunge into arctic water, or feeling as if a 'golden comb' is raking through your emotions during a sound bath, or treating our inner-child to the wholesome treat of a Ferris wheel or roller-skates. Or how's about a rope swing, kiddo?

Featuring luxurious writing you can sink into like a warm bath, this sent a thrill of electric possibility through me. It reminded me of the infinite choice of alcohol-free fun.

Best for: Pleasure-seekers who are no longer all about the sober chat, and want to roam all across the landscape. Or those feeling shifty, restless in longer-term sobriety, who want their horizons expanding.

Not for: Readers who want a book that's going to stay on the sober road. I'd guestimate that less than half of the content directly pertains to sobriety.

***

You'll notice something, when you look at the jackets of practically all of these books (or mine, for that matter). Many of the endorsement quotes are from 'competitors'.

And no, it's not because sober authors are part of some underground sorority or fraternity. Most of us have never even met. We have different publishers, agents, and zero to gain from lifting up each other's work. But we do it because it's the right thing to do.

We know there is *so much room*, in this sober realm. That it's already exploding, and will explode some more as the years roll by. We know that our book may not resonate with someone, but this other one might be the ladder they use to get themselves out of the manhole – the breadcrumb trail out of the woods.

To be clear, the reader does the work themselves to get sober; a book categorically cannot get you sober. Which is why, every time a reader sends me a beautiful letter crediting my words with their sobriety, I say, 'A book cannot do that for you. YOU did that, so take all the credit, my friend.'

<u>But books are maps.</u> Maps of how someone else found their way out of those godforsaken woods. Books can behave as cartographical signposts that assist the lost in getting un-lost. Which is why we big-up each other's work. We don't see each other as 'competitors'. We see each other as 'collaborators'.

Because: maps. We need lots of 'em.

STONE COLD VS SUNSHINE WARM TREE-BATHING

STONE COLD DRUNK TREE-BATHING

OCTOBER 2012

I start appreciating nature in my workaday lunchtimes. Staring at trees. Getting some fresh air.

At least, that's what I tell myself I'm doing. What I'm actually doing is: drinking in parks. At lunchtime.

It has previously been pubs, but pubs contain too many people for my liking, and my whimpering bank balance is no longer up to £6 glasses of chilled sauvignon blanc alongside my hangover-feeding lunch of a meatball wrap or a cheesy croissant, or whatever else is brown and cheap.

Eating has become a necessity, not a pleasure. Aged 32, I am increasingly affronted by my friends wanting to go for dinner, rather than just drinks. This dinner thing is so tiresome!

Take last night. '£15 for a sourdough pizza; you're having a laugh,' I snorted, throwing the menu down, and gesturing for the garçon so that I could order a £15 bottle of nasty house white instead.

I sat there defiantly not eating, choosing to spend my money on what mattered instead – the alcohol. I would later have a pizza procured from the newsagent freezer for £3. And feel like the winner in this equation. I have outwitted the sourdough pizza rip-off merchants!

Today, I feel like I am similarly outfoxing The Man, whoever he is. I tell myself drinking in a park is 'practically the same thing' as drinking in a pub, and a fuckofalot cheaper. What about all of my colleagues who go to The Green Man? I'm no different from them!

I buy an itty-bitty airplane-sized bottle of pink wine and decant it into a plastic coloured 'sports' bottle, which has a pop-up nozzle for speedy rehydration while running. For some reason the alcohol being pink makes it feel less harmful. Maybe this is why the whole 'pinking of gin' marketing has been so moon slingshot successful?

Right about now, given I had a bottle-and-a-half of wine last night, the last vestiges are starting to leave my system. This floods my nervous system with malevolent doom. The doom comes closer the longer I'm sober. It looms out of my hangover like a haunted castle sketching itself known into the fog.

I can't wait until the end of the working day any more. The doom is too much to bear. Luckily, I'm a wine-sneaking sleuth, a sleight-of-the-hand decanter; a blink-and-you'll-miss-it whizz.

So, I'm sitting there, in my natty little Oliver Bonas outfit (my silky top has hummingbirds on it, which I take as proof I am winning at life), reading Stylist, *munching on my brown food and drinking my pink drink that nobody knows about.*

Finished eating, I post a photo on Instagram of my colour-coded bookshelves, because everyone knows that you can't possibly be a fuck-up if you have colour-coded bookshelves.

Up bound two teenage girls, clearly on half term, both wearing tracksuits, and one holds a half-drunk bottle of vodka. They address me respectfully, as if I'm their teacher.

I'm staring intently at my phone, waiting for the likes.

Teen: 'We were wondering, Miss.'

Me: 'Hmmm?'

Teen: 'Do you want this?'

She offers the half-drunk vodka, smiles shyly.

Me: 'That? Why would I want that?'

Teen: 'Well, we saw that you was having a sly lunchtime drink, Miss, and we don't want the rest, so?'

I'm outraged and mortified, simultaneously. The cheek! Why are they watching me? But also – the shame! My charade has been penetrated by their wily teenage eyes.

Me: 'Oh, no thanks, I never drink vodka.'

(I do drink vodka, when in a tight spot. I just don't like it, but liking it is no longer the point. Demolishing the doom is).

The centrifugal force of my denial is moving my interpretation of reality further and further away from the centre of truth; the truth of how people see me. I tell myself they see a refined woman in a hummingbird top, who probably has colour-coded bookshelves at home (I do! Follow me on Instagram, girls!), when actually... they see something very different.

I have been kidding myself that my decanting, my drinking, is invisible. This is the day that I realise it's not. And suddenly I feel terribly, painfully visible.

SUNSHINE WARM SOBER TREE-BATHING

SEPTEMBER 2016

'Yeah, so there's this amazing Glens Red Squirrel Group thing, because red squirrels are so threatened due to the dastardly greys, and it turns out my distant cousin is the general secretary! Isn't that an absolute gas? Imagine being the general secretary of a squirrel protection group! It's so... woodsy! I'd love to read the minutes of their meetings.'

My boyfriend rolls his eyes.

And then I spiral off into a squirrel warzone skit where we arm red squirrels with tiny air rifles so they can protect themselves from the greys.

'What about tiny tanks too?' my boyfriend suggests.

'Yes!' I cry. 'They can wear little hard hats. And have hand grenades that look like acorns!'

I am in Glenariff Forest Park once more. Now three years sober, I appear to have become a squirrel enthusiast, just like my dad. Who knew sobriety came with automatic critter appreciation?! I am enchanted by this wild place that represents one of the last British boltholes for these threatened elf-eared creatures.

'How far's the restaurant?' he asks.

'I'm not entirely sure where we are,' I admit.

'I thought you said you have a natural sense of direction?'

'Every time I claim that, I get lost.'

He harumphs his way around the park. The enthusiasm drains from me. It's not unlike when you show someone your favourite film and their clenched reaction to it makes you unable to fully enjoy it yourself.

We finally find the restaurant. He dashes inside to order a pint and some food, while I linger outside. 'Just order me some chips and a Coke; I'll be in in a sec,' I say.

I trek back up the path and over the bridge to a glade we passed that has a magical quality to it. I feel sure that if I'm going to see a red squirrel, it'll be here. I nestle against the knot of a tree, tipping my face upwards to the canopy above and try and make myself perfectly still. I notice that the nature enchantment goes up, not down, when I'm utterly alone.

A flash of red! Is it? No, it's the scarlet cap of a red woodpecker. His pecking sounds almost man-made, like someone with a tiny pneumatic drill. I stay for a few more minutes, luxuriating in how small and gorgeously insignificant I feel among these towering fir and spruce spires.

I don't see a red squirrel. But it doesn't matter. Just the knowledge that they're there, hoarding nuts, gnawing on bark, scampering along branches, twitching their pointy elfin ears, polishing their tiny acorn grenades, is enough of a thrill.

The reds are shy, discreet and outnumbered. Not unlike the sobers. Who are out there too. Even when you can't see them.

IV: YEAR EIGHT

THE HOOKED FISH

(CONT'D)

The fish realised something transformative. That although the hook would always be close, it only held the power that the fish assigned to it. The fish no longer wanted to live in fear of the hook sneaking up on it. It no longer shrank at the sight of it, or felt ruled by its despotic sway.

So, the fish stopped swimming, turned and stared the hook down. And with that, the fish saw – once again – that the punch-pop of the neon was nothing but dye, and the feathers were nothing but fake fibres. The glint of the metal behind, veiled by the showgirl costumery, was now clearly visible to the fish.

The hook was not the dreamlike companion the fish had once been entranced by. It never had been, in fact. It still was – had always been – a pretty, seductive, ugly trap. The fish saw it for what it actually was, rather than what it pretended to be.

And so, the fish finally felt truly unhooked. Because the hook may well always be on the periphery of its vision. But the only way the hook could pluck the fish from its freedom again would be if the fish chose to go towards it.

And frankly, the fish had more bloody sense.

So it lived happily ever after instead.

YEAR EIGHT: THE CO-EXISTENCE OF TWO TRUTHS

'Whether you think you can, or think you can't, you're right'
Henry Ford

I'm now deep into my eighth year sober. Welcome to the 'ever after'. In which I've found that two seemingly contradictory truths can co-exist:

1.   I am not addicted now.

2.   If I were to re-start, I believe I would become addicted again.

I embody unhooked + the potential to be re-hooked. Freedom + vigilance. Those two jive together. What about you, if you're a long-term sober too? What do you embody?

There's a great ravine of difference between secure vigilance and forevermore fear. I know the hook's still there. But only I can choose to launch myself back upon it. To wrap my mouth around it. Nowadays, I don't believe that external elements have the ability to cast me back upon it. I've lived through infidelities, sudden grief, job loss, much trolling,* some significant break-ups and much more I haven't told you about, without wrapping my mouth back around the hook. So, I'm as sure as is humanly possible that I won't. Ever. Which feels lovely. If that's wrong, then I sure as hell don't want to be right.

---

* One misogynistic man commented 'Her future is feline' on a piece I wrote about being happily single. I want to put that on a T-shirt.

I recently sat around a table of love, with my family, to celebrate a male relative's milestone birthday. Speeches were made about how good and right this person is. And he is, he is good to his core. I sat there, an introvert with a speech to make. I chickened out – and then told him this directly, the next day...

Rewind to my 31st birthday. Having drunk approximately 22 units, I'd spent the hours of 1am to 3am whole-body sobbing because of the (spoken) fear I would be single for ever, but also the (unspoken) fear of my drinking.

Here's what my family member did, at the tender age of 21. Went out and bought a book for me entitled, *Everything is Going to be OK*. That small but astonishingly empathic gesture handed me a torch in a hopeless place. Even nine years on, every time I think about it, I feel moved.

***

These books on sobriety, of which this is my third, have been trying to do the same thing. To hand you a light source when you find yourself in a dark room. At the risk of quoting Rihanna, I wanted to show you some love and perhaps even a possible route *out* of the hopeless place. To say, 'everything is going to be OK' if you can just walk a little. One step. Then another.

If you're still there in that dark room of shame, whether sober or not, consider me there with you, with a torch. I know the GPS and every inch of that room, intimately. Our rooms contain different things, different memories, different actions, but I know how it feels to live there.

I know what it is to be walking through the supermarket and suddenly be plucked from banality, as if a stuffed animal grabbed by a giant claw, and dropped into a dark memory so shameful it makes your skin hurt.

As we've already discussed, that whole-body shame prickle recedes, with every good action, day and year you put between you and the shame. But it still has the power to air-drop you from a sunshine warm day into a stony, cold place. I know.

And I hope you feel that knowing and that companionship, wherever you may be in the process. I'm here, and I have a torch. I only wish I could hold your hands through the entire process.

I can't hold your hand through this. But! If you seek each other out, you can hold each other's hands instead. Because there are millions of us. You just need to go out and find each other, whether in meetings or on socials or in post-yoga chatter. Light up your own torches so that you can.

I probably won't continue to write books about sobriety, given to do so would start to require repetition, and it's up to the many other upcoming torch-bearers now. I have a big beautiful life to lead, even though, on the surface, it's actually pretty simple and modest. We are allowed to move beyond our addictions. To enjoy our newfound wild and precious freedom.

My sobriety is just a few months shy of the age of my niece. There she is, a walking, talking, plait-demanding, unicorn-horn-wearing manifestation of just how long it's been. How beautifully grown it now is. But just like her, it's not fixed or finished.

I'm not 'fixed'. But I'm not broken either. All of us sit someplace in between. I still say I'm in recovery because I think of recovery as this: uncovering who I was meant to be all along, before shit went south. Like the 'recovery' process of a document after a computer crashes. I'm still in the process of becoming – reclaiming – my best possible self. As we all are.

That doesn't mean I'm shooting towards becoming a *Gilmore Girl*-esque sweet, gingerbread person; I'm talking a person who's kind and good, but also a badass at self-care. Ideally, though, I would call it 'discovery' instead of 'recovery' these days. 'No thanks, I'm in discovery,' I would say to confused waiters with trays of fizz.

My opinions and beliefs about sobriety and recovery constantly evolve. I don't have the answers. Nobody does. And – more importantly – they're allowed to evolve. Pinning our beliefs to a board is like pinning a butterfly to a page. Beliefs that are fixed and immovable are essentially no longer living. No longer able to breathe, move or grow.

You can't possibly know how much it has helped me, to have the privilege of writing these books and having you read them. It's helped me illuminate things I wouldn't have otherwise seen or found. It's been a true honour to have you along for the ride as I have unpacked some of the darkest objects from my past, repacked and journeyed into the other side.

Thank you for being with me.

Go get 'em, tiger. I believe in you.

Much love,

Catherine

AFTERWORD

'If it makes you happy, then why the hell are you so sad?'

Sheryl Crow

EIGHT YEARS BEFORE SOBRIETY

SEPTEMBER 2005

I am still drunk. I know it.

My friends Kate and Suzy are coming to see my Shoreditch flat at 5pm. I will make them something that features cheese, pasta and chorizo, because I'm barely out of university and I still think that constitutes a dinner party.

Right now, it's 2pm and I feel like my head is in an ever-tightening vice. I need to sober up, shake this ennui and transform into hostess mode.

So, I go for a run. I've heard this works. I've tried it a lot. Sometimes it does. As I'm setting out, I pass a man.

'Cath. Oi, Cath!'

I have no idea who he is.

I stare at him blankly.

'Sorry, who...'

'You have no idea who I am, do you?'

'No, have we met?'

'Last Friday night, the lock-in. You really don't remember?'

I really don't. I am now aflame with shame.

He smirks. I have nothing to say to this man I do not know, so I walk off instead. I speed into a jog and then a sprint, trying to race from the horror that my body does things I don't remember.

I have to stop in the middle of the run to dry-retch into the grass. I sit down cross-legged and wipe my mouth. A window in my mind unclouds, as if I've fed money into a peepshow. I see the man looming over me in a hovel of a room bathed in grey dawn light. And the window clouds again.

That's it. That's all I have. The rest is lost. And I suspect I want it to stay lost.

I star shape on the grass and feel tears spill out of my eyes, even as I attempt to blink them back into my eye ducts. The ground beneath me feels stony, unforgiving, ice-cold.

I get home, shower, eat toast and feel marginally more human. I start drinking again while I wait for my friends to arrive. I am faux bright by the time they arrive. I mention nothing of the man from the memory peepshow. These are secrets I tuck away, because to share them would be to give the game away.

At one point, my mask slips and I forget to look happy. Suzy catches a glimpse of my real self. 'Are you OK?' she asks kindly, when Kate is in the toilet. 'Absolutely!' I respond too quickly, puffing myself up once more.

***

'Are you OK?' is my most dreaded question. Of course I'm OK!

I feel like a piñata, and 'Are you OK?' is the bat that threatens to split my fragile façade wide open. Inside there is no candy or toys; only regret, fags, booze and the phone numbers of many men.

I am not OK. I can't be trusted to look after myself. I feel unsafe. Hijacked.

My body does things I don't remember.

IN MY EIGHTH YEAR SOBER

OCTOBER 2020

I run and think, 'This is it'. This is what I was looking for – and never found – in drinking.

The relief from anxiety, the wild abandon, the affinity with the music, the pure pleasure, the 'Don't stop me now!' freedom I sought out on every dance floor. I pound the pavement in time with Moloko's 'The Time is Now' as I feel both 'at one' but also gloriously separate from all around me.

I bounce towards the kiss-me-quick capitalism of Palace Pier, with its gold-crossed-palm tarot reader in a gypsy caravan, its candy-floss-scented air and the Crazy Mouse roller-coaster (which you'd indeed have to be 'crazy' to go on, given it's a brokedown rustbucket that threatens to tip you into the biro-blue sea*).

I do my squats under the Victorian wrought-iron skeleton of the pier's underside. I watch huddled hooded teens smoke spice in an attempt to vacate their bodies. They're my people. I understand them. I get it. I've tried to touch the void of oblivion too. On an empty patch of promenade I sing along to Simple Minds' 'Alive and Kicking' and remember how I once tried to kill myself ever-so-slowly but, thankfully, failed.

I've been running into the wind; now I switch and run with the wind at my back. This newfound rocket-pack of wind power reminds me of the ease that we find the longer we go into sobriety. If we can only ignore the twang of our Achilles' heel and our lead-filled legs at the start, and focus instead on the fact we haven't felt this good all day – or indeed all of our lives – until now.

---

* Lawyers, chill your boots: I'm sure the Crazy Mouse roller-coaster is regularly serviced and as safe as roller-coasters can be :-)

I feel invincible, nimble, darting around the slow-honey boozehounds and blurred barflies spilling out of the seafront bars. Also my people. I doff my running cap to them. I watch the seagulls circling for chip-based quarry like fighter jets. I hear the moored boats' sails clanking like dinner plates in a rowdy boarding school.

I watch the glaze-eyed and deer-legged teens in the kissing booth of 'Shoosh', while listening to Skunk Anansie's 'Hedonism', I look at them and see the 19-year-old me.

Nights out were so often comparable to throwing myself upon a sacrificial altar of chance. Hoping I would come back alive. I resist the urge to kidnap the teens and take them sea-swimming instead.

I am no sobriety missionary. We have to discover this for ourselves. To try to convert others would not only be utterly futile, it would rob them of their own journey. Like the fabled stubborn horse, people can lead us to sobriety but they can't make us partake. It's up to us to do that.

As I sprint past the most hedonistic strip of bars, I feel free. I no longer feel like I am missing out on the one-more-bar, one-more-drink, one-more-something and we'll finally find it! search.

Sometimes, we did find it. We'd brush our fingers against it. Be in it for an instant and then – *snaps fingers* – it's gone. Where'd it go? What we seek never stays still; it's an ever-moving faerie that dances further and further into the night. That we would chase, instead of going home.

Nowadays, my endorphins are sponsored by exercise, loved ones and laughs, rather than Chenin Blanc. Others on the promenade know this too. I feel a kinship with the skaters, who bruise themselves joyously and film their tricks; the basketballers with their boom box and French rap; the volleyball team, who head home covered in sand, muscle-bashed, happy and tired.

I curve around the lagoon, upon which wakeboarders sometimes do tricks. The water sits waiting, serene, mirror-still; like an empty ballroom floor. I continue onto the nudist beach, my favourite flopping spot. The cheerful two-feet-tall 'Costa Del Bollocky' graffiti never fails to make me laugh. It sits next to the intensely middle-class wall announcement: 'I really dislike paella!'

I starfish on the floor like a sweat-angel in pebbles instead of snow. My view becomes an uninterrupted sky of denim blue. Tears come, but they're not sad ones. They're of relief, and I experience them often after the emotion-dislodging energy of a run. There's bliss in these tears.

I used to have to fake this bliss. Cheat my way into it. I looked for it in the bottom of thousands of bottles. Now the most ordinary moments have the power to make it. Even when I'm alone, I don't feel lonely, despite living alone (although my first puppy is imminent). I feel loved.

There are still times when a champagne cheers can twang me with awkwardness. I am an out-of-tune guitar plucked by the 'pop!' of the cork and the knowledge that I will not know where to put my hands or myself, while this group ritual happens without me.

The discordance lasts only three seconds, in a day otherwise full of comfort. This was not the case when I first got sober, fuck no. But now, the ratio of 'discomfort: comfort' has tipped overwhelmingly, ridiculously so towards the comfort. Maybe you need to get incredibly uncomfortable in order to learn how to feel comfortable? Maybe you need to practise not fleeing your own skin in order to feel radical comfort within it? I think so.

There is no such thing as having it all, though. As with anything in life that requires great change and sacrifice – a promotion, a baby, buying a house, emigrating – it's a barter. You cash something in to get something else.

You can't be both the down-with-the-staff employer and the respected boss; you can't have both the freedom of renting and the security of buying. And you can't have both the blur of drunk and the clarity of sober. The challenge lies in creating an existence that you no longer need or want to blur. That you can live in, pin-sharp.

I've found that what you get with sobriety is so much more valuable, more precious, than what you give. You leave your friends at the bar because soda water doesn't make you want to stay out until 1am, and miss out on some of the banter they reminisce about the next day...they skinny-dipped and are now calling themselves 'The Night Swimmers'! But on the way home you see a shooting star.

You give, you get. And, as with so many things, your investment adjusts the rewards. The more effort you put into cultivating a bloom in sobriety, the more verdant it will become.

What I had before was confinement. It was small, ever-shrinking and tethered to my dependence on a drug that was systematically destroying me. What I have now is huge, ever-expanding and untethered.

I don't hold the tears back. I let them flow. A saddle-brown elderly nudist looks slightly concerned about me, but he needn't be. He waves enthusiastically at me, his testicles waggling. I wave back. He reclines, reassured.

I shut my eyes. The blazing-ball sunshine is visible even through my eyelids. I feel the warmth.

This is it. This is what I was looking for in that.

I feel safe. Loved. Like I belong. Finally.

I'm safe.

SOURCES

INTRODUCTION

Relapse rates after three years of abstinence: Michael L. Dennis, Mark A. Foss and Christy K. Scott, 'An Eight-Year Perspective on the Relationship Between the Duration of Abstinence and Other Aspects of Recovery', published online by ResearchGate, December 2007.

All 2020 NHS data: 'Statistics on alcohol, England, Part 4: Drinking behaviours among adults', published by NHS Digital, 5 February 2020.

A third of millennials planned to host a teetotal Christmas; half said they would not drink during Christmas dinner: Richard Jenkins, 'Third of millennials will host a teetotal Christmas this year', published online in the *Independent*, 9 December 2020.

No/low alcohol beer sales up 30 per cent since 2016: '"Nolo beer" sales rocket thanks to young teetotallers', published online by the BBC, 12 March 2020.

Lockdown drinking stats from Alcohol Change UK: Lucy Holmes, blog 'Drinking during lockdown: headline findings', published by Alcohol Change UK, April 2020.

Glass that holds an entire bottle of Prosecco banned: Emma Reed, 'Prosecco is a drink not a personality', published online in *Metro*, 9 December 2020.

Advertising Standards Authority (ASA) bans posts by Scottish Gin Society: 'Watchdog bans gin ads after complaints upheld', published online in the *Glasgow Evening Times*, 5 September 2018.

Globally, deaths from alcohol are increasing: 'Alcohol use and burden for 195 countries and territories, 1990–2016: a systematic analysis for the Global Burden of Disease Study 2016', published online in *The Lancet*, volume 392, issue 10152, pages 1015–35, 22 September 2018.

YEAR FIVE: THE NEW MORAL NORMAL

70 per cent cheated because they were 'drunk and not thinking clearly': Dylan Selterman, Justin R. Garcia and Irene Tsapelas, 'Motivations for Extradyadic Infidelity Revisited', published online in *The Journal of Sex Research*, pages 273–86, 15 December 2017.

2016 study into 800+ university students finds problem drinking is a 'significant' predictor of infidelity: Steven M. Graham, Sesan Negash, Nathaniel M. Lambert and Frank D. Fincham, 'Problem Drinking and Extradyadic sex in young adult relationships', *Journal of Social and Clinical Psychology*, volume 35, number 2, pages 152–70, 2016.

23 per cent of Brits shoplifted as kids: cited in 'Quarter of Brits have shoplifted', published online by YouGov, 16 March 2020.

Quote from 2014 study: H. Garavan, K. L. Brennan, R. Hester and R. Whelan, 'The Neurobiology of Successful Abstinence', published online by PubMed (PMCID: PMC3706547), 1 August 2014.

Hangovers are the top reason we phone in sick: Anthony Bruce, 'Three ways to find a remedy for costly "sickies"', *PWC UK blog*, 2 July 2014.

Morning-after calculator drink/drive calculator: *www.morning-after.org.uk*

GIN/SPIN

Here are examples of alcohol-slogan sportswear and sports gear:
Gin and Yin: *https://www.moreyoga.co.uk/whats-on/gin-yin*

Spin and Gin: *https://www.digmefitness.com/events/details/spin-n-gin*

Tough Mudder: 'World's Best Mud Run and Obstacle Course', *https://www.toughmudder.co.uk/articles/brewdog-is-your-2019-tough-mudder-uk-finisher-drink*
And 'Will there be Alcohol', *https://www.toughmudderaushelp.zendesk.com/hc/en-us/articles/115003078791-Will-there-be-alcohol*

Pinot Pilates: *https://www.pinotpilates.com.au*

Wine and Yoga: *https://www.yogaboutiqueuk.com/wine-yoga*

Ronnie O'Sullivan quote: 'Rehab was the moment my career truly started', published online in *Eurosport UK*, 23 April 2020.

Andy Fordham once drank so much playing darts he'd have still failed a breath test three days later: article by Mike Walters, published online in the *Mirror/Sport*, 8 January 2016.

2019 study on drinking wine equivalent to smoking cigarettes: Stephen Matthews, 'Risk of getting cancer from drinking just one bottle of wine is the same as smoking up to 10 cigarettes a week', published in the *MailOnline*, 28 March 2018.

BMA and National Institutes for Health and Clinical Excellence (NICE) call for a ban on alcohol sports sponsorship: Ben Cooper, 'Alcohol sponsorship – last orders for sports sponsorship', published online in *Reuters Events*, 17 December 2009.

France and Norway have banned alcohol sponsorship of sporting events, while Italy has severely restricted it. Plus research on rejections and bans of tabacco and alcohol sponsorship: Timothy Chambers, 'Unhealthy sponsorship of sport', *British Medical Journal,* 4 December 2019.

Russia reverses ban on alcohol advertising during World Cup 2018: article by Mark Lammey, published online in the *Moscow Times*, 5 July 2014.

Scottish women's football will reject alcohol or gambling sponsors: article published online in *BBC Sport*, 1 October 2018.

Egyptian player refuses Budweiser-sponsored award: article on goalkeeper Mohamed El-Shenawy, published online in *Reuters/ Sport*, 16 June 2018.

DRINKING/DEBT

Meta-analysis which found those with debt are 2.68 times more likely to exhibit AUD than those without: Thomas Richardson, Peter Elliot and Ronald Roberts, 'The relationship between personal unsecured debt and mental and physical health: a systematic review', published online by PubMed (PMID 24121465), 10 September 2013.

IN BED WITH BIG ALCOHOL

Alcohol taxation made the government duty between £10.5 and £12.1 billion in the past five years: 'UK Alcohol Duty Statistics', published online by Gov.UK, 29 May 2020.

Public Health England says alcohol harm costs £21 billion a year minimum: Dr Robyn Burton, Clive Henn, Don Lavoie, Rosanna O'Connor, Clare Perkins, Kate Sweeney, Felix Greaves, Brian Ferguson, Caryl Beynon, Annalisa Belloni, Virginia Musto, Professor John Marsden, Professor Nick Sheron, Alanna Wolff and staff at PHE, 'The Public Health Burden of Alcohol and the Effectiveness and Cost-Effectiveness of Alcohol Control Policies', published online by Gov.UK, Public Health, gateway no. 2016490, December 2016.

France cancels Dry January: 'Dry January? France says "Non" as winemakers cry foul', published online by *France 24*, 21 November 2019.

New York Times exposes scandal on federal agency courting Big Alcohol's money: article by Roni Caryn Rabin, published online in *The New York Times*, 17 March 2018.

$100 million study is then axed after an investigation: Lucy A Taylor, 'Twenty things I wish I'd known when I started my PhD', published online in *Nature*, 6 November 2020.

Drinkaware website quotes and details of their campaigns: screenshots from Drinkaware website, 29 October 2020, 6 November 2020 and 11 December 2020.

2013 report 'Be Aware of Drinkaware': Jim McCambridge, Kypros Kypri, Peter Miller, Ben Hawkins and Gerard Hastings, published online by PubMed (PMCID PMC3992826), 28 October 2013.

Portman Group statement and 'risks': 'Putting the "risks" of alcohol consumption into context', published online by the Portman Group, 16 April 2019.

British alcohol-specific deaths in 2017 totalled 21 deaths per day: 'Alcohol-specific deaths in the UK: registered in 2017', published online by the Office for National Statistics, 4 December 2019.

Royal Society for Public Health calls the public blind spot around the risks of drinking an 'awareness vacuum': Katie Silver, 'Calls for mandatory health information on alcohol labels', published on *BBC News online*, 27 January 2018.

Letter signed by 25 health leaders: 'AHA response to the news that alcohol producers will no longer be advised to display the drinking guidelines labels', published online by Alcohol Health Alliance, 11 October 2017.

April 2020 advice from the World Health Organization: cited in 'Alcohol does not protect against Covid 19; access should be restricted during lockdown', published online by WHO/Europe, 14 April 2020.

The impacts of outlawing alcohol sales in South Africa and some Mexican states: from an episode of *Business Daily*, adapted for text by Bryan Lufkin, published online by *BBC Global*.

Nielsen 67 per cent surge in alcohol sales in March 2020: cited in article by Jonathan Eley, published online by the *Financial Times*, 31 March 2020.

Americans are advised by CDC to avoid alcohol during Thanksgiving/ in general: Marlene Lenthang, 'CDC holiday guidelines tell Americans not to sing, listen to loud music or drink alcohol to prevent the spread of COVID-19', published in the *MailOnline*, 18 November 2020.

MPs drink more than average citizen: Rahul Rao, Ioannis Bakolis, Jayati Das Munshi, Daniel Poulter, Nicole Votruba and Graham Thornicroft, 'Alcohol consumption of UK members of parliament: cross-sectional survey', published online in *BMJ Open*, 1 March 2020.

Dr Dan Poulter quote in the *Guardian*: Toby Helm, 'Last orders! Report calls time on boozy Westminster culture', published online in the *Guardian*, 7 March 2020.

THE PROBLEMATIC LANGUAGE AROUND THE PROBLEM

Jon Hamm reveals he went to rehab for alcoholism ahead of final *Mad Men* season: article published online in the *Guardian*, 25 March 2015.

More 'punitive measures' recommended for 'abusers' rather than those with 'use disorders': John F. Kelly and Cassandra M. Westerhoff, 'Does it matter how we refer to individuals with substance-related conditions? A randomized study of two commonly used terms', published online by PubMed (PMID 20005692), 14 December 2009.

Refuge quote from interview with Buddhist teacher Noah Levine: Joan Duncan Oliver, 'The Suffering of Addiction', published online in *Tricycle*, 26 September 2014.

2018 study into the efficacy of AA and AA alternatives: Sarah E. Zemore, Camillia Lui, Amy Mericle, Jordana Hemberg and Lee Ann Kaskutas, 'A longitudinal study of the comparative efficacy of Women for Sobriety, LifeRing, SMART Recovery, and 12-step groups for those with AUD', published online by the *Journal of Substance Abuse Treatment*, 17 February 2018.

Bill W.'s 1946 essay for *The Grapevine*: Bill, 'Who is a Member of AA?', *The Grapevine*, 1946

National Institutes of Health on avoiding terms 'addict' and 'alcoholic': 'Words matter – terms to use avoid when talking about addiction', published online by National Institutes for Health, 28 January 2021.

Six papers regarding the stigma that accompanies 'alcoholic' or 'addict'. Half also mention that the stigma can deter people from seeking help.
1 James C. Dean and Gregory A. Poremba, 'The Alcoholic Stigma and the Disease Concept', published online by the American Psychological Association, 3 July 2009.
2 Memorandum 'Changing the Language of Addiction', from the Office of National Drug Policy Control to Heads of Department during President Obama's administration, 9 January 2017.
3 W. White, 'The rhetoric of recovery advocacy: An essay on the power of language', *Let's Go Make Some History: Chronicles of the New Addiction Recovery Advocacy Movement*, Johnson Institute and Faces and Voices of Recovery, pages 37–76, 2006.
4 John F. Kelly, Richard Saitz and Sarah Wakeman, 'Language, Substance Use Disorders, and Policy: The Need to Reach Consensus on an "Addictionary"', published online in *Alcoholism Treatment Quarterly*, 8 January 2016.

5 Georg Schomerus, Michael Lucht, Anita Holzinger, Herbert Matschinger, Mauro G Carta and Matthias C. Angermeyer, 'The Stigma of Alcohol Dependence Compared with Other Mental Disorders: A Review of Population Studies', published online in *Alcohol and Alcoholism*, volume 46, issue 2, pages 105–12, March–April 2011.

6 Steve Matthews, Robyn Dwyer and Anke Snoek, 'Stigma and Self-Stigma in Addiction', published online in the *Journal of Bioethical Inquiry*, 3 May 2017.

Example of a scientific addiction journal changing its lexicon to person-first language: Lauren M. Broyles, Ingrid A. Binswanger, Jennifer A. Jenkins, Deborah S. Finnell, Babalola Faseru, Alan Cavaiola, Marianne Pugatch and Adam J. Gordon, 'Confronting Inadvertent Stigma and Pejorative Language in Addiction Scholarship: A Recognition and Response', published online by *PubMed*, (PMCID PMC6042508), 12 July 2018.

YEAR SIX: WE REPEAT WHAT WE DON'T REPAIR

Having a tough time in childhood means you are seven times more likely to become addicted to alcohol later in life: James A. Reavis, Jan Looman, Kristina A. Franco and Briana Rojas, 'Adverse Childhood Experiences and Adult Criminality: How Long Must We Live before We Possess Our Own Lives?', *The Permanente Journal*, Spring 2013, 44–8.

About the CDC – Kaiser Permanente ACE study: 'Relationship of Childhood Abuse and Household Dysfunction to Many of the Leading Causes of Death in Adults', published online by Centers for Disease Control and Prevention, US, April 2020.

2018 study into childhood trauma and elevated empathy: David M. Greenberg, Simon Baron-Cohen, Nora Rosenberg, Peter Fonagy and Peter J. Rentfrow, 'Elevated empathy in adults following childhood trauma', published online in *Plos One*, 3 October 2018.

KIDS: UNDERAGE DRINKING MEANS HIGHER ADDICTION

Those who start drinking before age 15 are four times more likely to become addicted later: press release published online by National Institute on Alcohol Abuse and Alcoholism (NIAAA), 14 January 1998.

29 per cent of 18–24-year-olds don't drink: 'Nearly 30% of young people in England do not drink, study finds', published online in the *Guardian*, 10 October 2018.

NUS survey finds a fifth of undergraduates have never drunk, but 70 per cent feel pressured to: article by Zahra Iqbal, published online in *The Gryphon*, 10 October 2018.

Alcohol responsible for one in four deaths among 16–24-year-olds: 'Fact sheet on alcohol consumption, alcohol-attributable harm and alcohol responses in European Union Member States, Norway and Switzerland', published online by the World Health Organization, 14 November 2018.

WHY ARE PREGNANT WOMEN STILL TOLD 'ONE WON'T HURT'?

Four in ten pregnant Brits drink during pregnancy: Kat Lay, 'Britons among the world's worst for drinking during pregnancy', published online in *The Times*, 20 January 2017.

BMJ article: 'Evidence for potential harms of light drinking in pregnancy "surprisingly" limited', published online in *BMJ Open* and the *Guardian*, 11 September 2017.

ACTUAL CRAVINGS VS UNCOMFORTABLE EMOTIONS

Humans of New York quote: from 'I wish I'd partied a little less', cited on *www.humansofnewyork.com/post/78679045171/i-wish-id-partied-a-little-less-people-always*.

Gut–brain connection: article published online in *Harvard Health Publishing*, March 2012.

THE TERRIBLE TWINS: BOOZE & COCAINE

2015 study finds alcohol use increases cocaine craving: Katherine R. Marks, Erika Pike, William W. Stoops and Craig R. Rush, 'Alcohol administration increases cocaine craving but not cocaine cue attentional bias', published online by PubMed (PMCID PMC4562057), 1 September 2016.

UNREPORTED BENEFIT OF SOBRIETY #117: HIGHER FERTILITY

Danish study of fertility in 6,120 women: Ellen M. Mikkelsen, Anders H. Riis, Lauren A. Wise, Elizabeth E. Hatch, Kenneth J. Rothman, Heidi T. Cueto and Henrik Toft Sørensen, 'Alcohol consumption and fecundability: prospective Danish cohort study', published online by PubMed (PMCID PMC5007353), 31 August 2016.

Danish study of 430 couples: Tina Kold Jensen, Niels Henrik I. Hjollund, Tine Brink Henriksen, Thomas Scheike, Henrik Kolstad, Aleksander Giwercman, Erik Ernst, Jens Peter Bonde, Niels E. Skakkebæk and Jørn Olsen, 'Does moderate alcohol consumption affect fertility? Follow up study among couples planning first pregnancy', published online by *PubMed* (PMCID PMC28642), 22 August 1998.

Harvard study on fertility during IVF: Brooke V. Rossi, Katharine F. Berry, Mark D. Hornstein, Daniel W Cramer, Shelley Ehrlich and Stacey A. Missmer, 'Effect of Alcohol Consumption on In Vitro Fertilization', article available on Harvard University Digital Access to Scholarship, January 2011.

Guardian quotes Tony Rutherford: Ian Sample, 'Alcohol hinders having a baby through IVF, couples warned', published online in the *Guardian*, 20 October 2009.

ANXIETY SOOTHING SUPERSIZED

20 per cent of the socially anxious become addicted to alcohol: cited in 'Social Anxiety Disorder and Alcohol Abuse', online by the Anxiety and Depression Association of America.

YEAR SEVEN: ASKING FOR WHAT WE NEED

2008 study on surprise windfall and spending it on others: Elizabeth W. Dunn, Lara B. Aknin and Michael I. Norton, 'Spending Money on Others Promotes Happiness', published online in *Science*, volume 319, issue 5870, pages 1687–8, 21 March 2008.

Altruism activates the striatum: Megan M. Filkowski, R. Nick Cochran and Brian W. Haas 'Altruistic behavior: mapping responses in the brain', published online by *PubMed* (PMCID PMC5456281), 4 November 2016.

The Crane Wife URL: *https://www.theparisreview.org/blog/2019/07/16/the-crane-wife.* C.J. Hauser, published online, 16 July 2019.

Eric Clapton quote: from an interview on 9 October 2007, 'What I've Learned', published online in *Esquire*, 6 October 2014.

WHY ARE DOCTORS MORE LIKELY TO BE BIG DRINKERS?

Doctors three times more likely and lawyers higher likelihood too: 'Alarm at growing addiction problems among professionals', Tracy Mcveigh, published online in the *Guardian*, 13 November 2011.

For higher earners drinking more: 'Statistics on alcohol, England, Part 4: Drinking behaviours among adults', published by *NHS Digital*, 5 February 2020.

THE ANTI-JOY OF UNEXPECTED TRIGGERS

£158 million in extra alcohol sales in 2017 heatwave: Sarah Butler, 'Sport and sunshine fuel surge in UK supermarket alcohol sales', published online in the *Guardian*, 25 July 2017.

2019 clinical study into PMS and anger: Havva Yesildere and Fatma Basar, 'The relationship between premenstrual syndrome and anger' published online by PubMed (PMCID PMC6500841), 2019.

2017 study into PMT and increased alcohol seeking/craving: The University of Illinois at Chigaco, 'Higher estrogen levels linked to increased alcohol sensitivity in brain's "reward center"', published online in *ScienceDaily*, 7 November 2017.

Example of British police force linking full moon with rising arrests: Fred Attewill, 'Police link full moon to aggression', published online in the *Guardian*, 5 June 2007.

INDEX

A

Abominable anecdote 226
accountability 30, 244
ACEs 124–44, 149–50, 280
addiction 91–2, 202
 accepting reality of 96
 addictive personality 68–9
 always? 240–1
 described 23–6
 as disease? 194–5
 genetic link 165–6
 as identity 102
 universal experience of 243–4
advertising, *see* marketing
affective empathy 137
aggression 82, 136, 248, 284
'alcohol abuse' phrasing 92–3
Alcohol Change UK 12
alcohol-use disorder (AUD) 60, 93, 94, 96, 105
Alcoholics Anonymous (AA) 41, 94, 96–7
anger 137–9, 230–2
anti-joy 218–27, 284
anxiety 3, 17, 48–9, 62, 68, 87, 111, 131, 153, 165–6, 168–70, 177, 223, 269, 283
 caffeinated 198
 soothing 196–200
arrogance 216–17
awareness vacuum 74

B

Baby Boomers 3, 11, 12
backpack of rocks 140–2
Big Alcohol 11–13, 70–8, 92, 252
binge-drinking 4, 11–12, 12, 21, 43,
46, 153, 177, 213
BIPOC 247–50
birthdays 106–9
BMA 57, 74
BMJ 57–8, 77, 156, 157
boozehounds vii, 5, 11, 34, 67, 183–9
boundaries 10, 79–83
Bowling, Dr Susan 198
brain function 20, 30–1, 61, 66, 99, 101, 111, 121, 149, 154–5, 165, 171, 176, 194–9, 202–3, 222, 229, 252
 and addiction 23–4, 240–1, 284
 logical vs lizard 226
 PFC 35
 subcortical 29
brain mapping 283
branding 53–8, 207
break-ups 209–11
breakfast drinking 12, 112, 154–5
breastfeeding 14, 116, 158–9
Buddhify 199
Buddhism 96, 171, 197, 199, 223, 232, 278
'butterflies' 171
button-pressing 139–40

C

CDC 77, 124, 278, 280
celebrities 233–9
Chamber of Shame 10, 28, 39–42
champagne breakfast 154–5
cheating, in relationships 31–2, 171
childhood trauma 14, 93, 124–38, 140–4, 247, 280
cirrhosis 14, 95, 212, 214
cliff edge GPS 245–6, 264

Club Soda 86
clubbing 130, 145, 150, 233
cocaethylene (CE) 174
cocaine 14, 21, 31, 112, 172–8, 282
confirmation bias 56, 244–5
conflicting messaging 157
connection 134–5
courage 97, 168, 242, 243, 254
Covid-19 76, 145, 225
craving 169–71, 219
Crow, Sheryl 267
'cut back and feel better' campaign 73

D
debt 60–7
deck-chair rearranging 100–1
delinquency 36–8, 150
detachment 116, 135, 139, 189, 191
detox 52–3, 55, 58
Didion, Joan 42
diet 40, 66, 126
difficult emotions 169–71
disingenuous empathy 216
doctors, heavy drinking of 212–17
dog-sitting 179–82
drink-cheating 254
drink-driving 43, 190, 214, 254, 274
drink-free days 73
Drink? (Nutt) 24, 76, 253–4
Drinkaware 72–6, 92
Dry January 13, 71, 276

E
early stress 128–32
eating disorders 126
echoes 134–5
El-Shenawy, Mohamed 58
emotion:
    'catching' 136
    vs craving 169–70
    uncomfortable 170–1

empathy 135–7, 191, 216
encouragement 71–5, 84, 96, 104, 114, 139, 156, 208, 244
entitlement 216–17
Eyre, Amanda 255

F
FARE 76
Farrell, Colin 233
Fat Tony 234
Fédération Addiction 71
fertility 192–3, 282
festivals 110–14
50 Cent 237
finances 60–7
flirting 84, 85, 145–6
Ford, Henry 263
Fordham, Andy 56
freedom 263–5
freeloading 37, 63–4
friendships 29, 167, 190–1, 267–8
Frith, Dr Chris 199
frontal-lobe activity 35
further reading 5, 251–6

G
Gay and Sober 86
gay community 14, 84–6, 168
Generation X 3, 12
Generation Z 3, 50, 114, 151–4
genetics 165–6
Gibran, Kahlil 136
Gollum anecdote 121–2
government revenue 70
Grace, Annie 159
Grisel, Dr Judith 23, 24, 29, 61, 68, 104, 125, 149–50, 165–6, 174, 194–5, 240
group-sharing 14, 44–6
Groves, Mark 83
gut–brain connection 282
gut instinct 171

H

hangover 22, 35, 38, 39–40, 44–5, 45, 48, 61, 80, 86, 116–19, 166, 178–9, 209, 213, 221–6, 257–8, 274
  allies 185–6
  denial 186–7
  'eye' 235
  long-term 237–9
  therapy 143–4
Hanson, Dr Rick, 197–8
hard drugs 14, 21, 31, 112, 172–8, 190, 282
Health 198
heavy drinking 115, 212–17
'helper's high' 202
'Home and Dry' campaign 73
'The Hooked Fish' (Gray) 7–8, 262

I

identity 96–102, 168
ill health 225–7
inhibition 19, 29, 85, 177, 196
interpretation 41, 169–71, 198, 259
intervention 188–9
intoxicated masculinity 167
IVF 192–3, 282, 283

J

judgement 5, 43, 117, 118, 139, 154, 158–9, 183–4, 210, 234, 255
'just an addict' narrative 242–3

K

Kaiser Permanente 124, 280
kindness 199
King Kong anecdote 13, 32–4
Kolk, Bessel van der 133

L

labelling 96–105, 244
labour, drinking during 159
Lancet Psychiatry i
Langley-Obaugh, Christine 128

language 92–105
  importance of 92–4
  'people first' 101–2
Latour, Nathalie 71
Lewis, Dr Julia 23, 24, 68, 77, 105, 165, 195, 241
Lewis, Dr Marc 23, 24, 68–9, 104, 124, 126, 165, 194, 240
LGBTQIA community 14, 168
Libaire, Jardine 255
LifeRing 96
liquid courage 47
lived experience 15, 97, 244–5
liver disease 14, 95, 212, 215
loneliness 216–17
long-term sobriety 14
Loper, Brendan 137
loving-kindness 199
low-alcohol, *see* no/low-alcohol

M

McKowen, Laura 189, 254–5
manipulation 4, 139, 157
marketing 4, 12–13, 20, 53–5, 57–8, 71–2, 91–2, 115, 116–17, 117–18, 220–1, 238, 253, 258, 273, 275
masculinity 167–8
MDMA 31, 190
meat industry 12, 29, 257
medical profession, heavy drinking within 212–17
meditation 32, 185, 196, 197, 199, 223, 251
Memoirs of an Addicted Brain (Lewis) 23
men's health 167–8
mental health 12, 14, 93–4, 120, 137, 153
metaphorical value 61
micro-aggression 136, 248
Millennials 3, 12, 32, 273
moderation 73, 121–2
moral compass 28–9

morning after 17, 43, 179, 186, 274
munchies 132

N

narcissism 40, 80, 138, 199
National Institute of Health (NIH)
101
National Institute on Alcohol Abuse
and Alcoholism 71
National Union of Students (NUS)
152
needs 202–8
neglect 126–7, 138, 171
NHS 11, 56, 71, 74, 133, 156, 157,
203, 212, 212–14
NICE 57
Nielsen 77, 278
no/low-alcohol 12, 14, 25, 273
non-labelling 96–100
'none is best' advice 156
normies 94–5
Nutt, Dr David 24, 68, 70, 72, 105,
165, 174, 194, 240, 253–4

O

obsessive compulsive disorder
(OCD) 126
ocean-going 47–51
off-licences 76–7
offloading 99
One Year No Beer 216
online recovery 96
The Only One in the Room 247, 250
opiates 174
O'Sullivan, Ronnie 55–6

P

parenting 115–20, 254
partying 61, 87–90, 91, 235
passive-aggressive 82
Perry, Philippa 144
phrasing 92–4
Pilates 54, 55

pivoting 102–3
PMT/PMS 219, 222–5, 284
post-birth recovery plan 116–17
post-natal depression (PND) 14,
116–17
Poulter, Dr Dan 77–8
pre-frontal cortex (PFC) 35
pre-menstrual tension/syndrome
(PMT/PMS), *see* PMT/PMS
predisposition 68–98, 124, 126, 165
pregnancy 156–61
procrastination, 14, 219, 221–2
Prohibition 76
psychosis 177
Public Health England (PHE) 70

Q

Queers without Beers (QWB) 86
Quit Like a Woman (Whitaker) 90,
252–3

R

racial identity 247–50
Refuge Recovery 96
R-E-S-P-E-C-T 175
retox 52–3, 55
Robbins, Laura Cathcart 247–50
In The Rooms 94, 101–2, 247–50
Rosen, Ellis 137
Royal Society for Public Health 74
Rumi 91
Rutherford, Tony 193

S

Sandberg, Sheryl 222
Scottish Gin Society 13
second childhood 132–3
Sedaris, David 237–8
self-destruction 24, 216–17
self-fulfilling prophecy 244–5
self-identification 95
self-loathing 41, 48, 138
self-parenting 142–4

sexual abuse 140–1, 177
sexual activity 14, 17, 31–2, 171, 192–3, 228, 282
shell charities 72–4
Sheron, Dr Nick 95
shoplifting 34–5, 274
sick notes 38–9, 44–6, 274
Siegel, Dr Michael 71–2
Singer, Michael A. 139
sleep 24, 29, 36, 48, 107, 119, 121, 127, 132–3, 164, 173–5, 177, 179–80, 226
    deprivation 40, 112, 117, 159, 212–14
sleight of hand 92–3
sloganising 92–4
smoking 12, 56, 92, 93, 202, 242, 275
sober adopters 152
sober-curiosity 17–18
sober dating 237
sober flirting 145–6
sobering up 84–6
sobriety, sustaining 9–10, 265, 269–72
sponsorship 56–9
stealing 34–5, 274
Step 5 (AA) 41
stigma 96, 98, 101–5, 279, 280
stone cold drunk, vs sunshine warm sober 47–51, 88–90, 106–14, 162–4, 179–82, 209–11, 230–2, 257–60
stone cold sober, described 3
Stonewall Inn 84, 85
stress 128–32
subtext 51, 95, 142, 186
summer 162–4, 219–21
sunshine warm sober:
    defined 3
    vs stone cold drunk 47–51, 88–90, 106–14, 209–11, 257–60
synaptic superhighways 194

T
Tempest 96
'The Temple of Boon' (Gray) 19–22
therapy hangover 143–4
Thorn, Michael 76
tobacco 12, 57, 58, 62, 252 (*see also* smoking)
tough love 187
Tough Mudder 54
trash-talk 142–3
tree-bathing 257–60
triggers 139, 218–29, 241, 284
12-step groups 96
two truths 263–5

U
underage drinking 147–52
The Unexpected Joy of Being Sober (Gray) 4, 5
unexpected triggers 14, 218–29, 284
universal experience 243–4
upper/downer effect 174

V
Vale, Jason 100
vigilance 263–5

W
W, Bill 97
We Are the Luckiest (McKowen) 253–4
wellness industry 14, 53
Which? 63
Whitaker, Holly 90, 252–3
WHO 72, 76
whole-body sobbing 264
Women for Sobriety (WFS) 96

ALSO AVAILABLE FROM CATHERINE GRAY

THE *SUNDAY TIMES* BESTSELLER

'Jaunty, shrewd and convincing'
The Sunday Telegraph

the

unexpected

joy of

being

sober

'Admirably honest, light, bubbly
and remarkably rarely annoying'
The Guardian

catherine gray

Also
available as
an ebook and
audiobook

Also
available as
an ebook

THE SUNDAY TIMES BESTSELLING AUTHOR OF
THE UNEXPECTED JOY OF BEING SOBER

catherine gray

the

unexpected

joy of

being

sober

journal

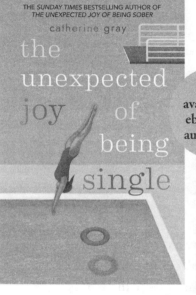

THE *SUNDAY TIMES* BESTSELLING AUTHOR OF
THE UNEXPECTED JOY OF BEING SOBER

catherine gray

the
unexpected
joy   of
       being
       single

Also
available as
ebook and
audiobook

the
unexpected
joy of
the
ordinary

CATHERINE GRAY
The *Sunday Times*
Bestselling
Author

ACKNOWLEDGEMENTS

A colossal thanks to the 50+ readers who contributed to this book, devoting their time, intelligence, humour and commendable honesty. I am honoured to have heard your stories; they are hands-down my favourite parts of this book.

Bottomless gratitude to my readers in general, who continue to read, review, big-up and gift my books. Receiving a beautiful DM or email from a reader is something that will never get old. I only wish I could meet you all for a tea sometime, because you all strike me as straight-up legends.

My agent Rachel Mills is someone whom I now never want to be without; a backflippin', kind, parkourin', funny literary genius whose feedback and guidance always makes my work better. The team at Aster and Octopus have become an expected joy to work with, especially my generous, warm and whip-smart publisher Stephanie Jackson (whose patience during the 'subtitle saga' was unparalleled ;-), the subtle-knife wonder of Pauline Bache, press-wrangler Karen Baker who deserves all the awards, digital marketing whizz Matthew Grindon, Kevin Hawkins and his deft sales team, and last but definitely not least, Yasia Williams-Leedham, who has overseen yet another cover that I want to hang on my wall.

Big-up to very talented designer Tamara Vodden, who is responsible for the gorgeous sunflowers on this jacket and the resting swallow (a neat echo of the flying swallow of *The Unexpected Joy of Being Sober*). To Millie for endless support and the voles. For Kate, who helped me juggle and organise the many, many case studies and without whom this aspect would have been impossible. To Niall and Fearne, who very kindly turned around endorsement quotes in an incredibly short timeframe. And gratitude to Lali and Galina, whose outrageously generous housewarming gift has given me the ability to focus in any hubbub. On that note, to Platf9rm, for creating a co-working space that does indeed make work wonderful.

My experts are utterly invaluable in this process, so a huge thank you goes out to Dr Julia Lewis and Dr Marc Lewis, for coming with me for another rodeo, as well as Professor David Nutt and Dr Judith Grisel, for joining me for the first time. Your illuminating, myth-busting and searing insights were fascinating to listen to and write up. Plaudits to Laura Cathcart Robbins, who wrote a brilliant and important essay and was a pleasure to deal with at every turn. And Joanne Bradford, for writing a piece which I was sad to have to lose, but grateful to get.

A heartfelt thanks to my first readers, in no particular order – Sarah Linford, Kate Faithfull, Seb Royle, Aoife Crehan, Andy Mac, Jamie Lissow, Laurie McAllister, Benji Lamb and Ion Tsakalis. Your feedback and time is much appreciated. You truly helped me make the book better.

And finally, I am endlessly grateful for my wonderful friends, family and loved ones, many of whom I haven't been able to see for a year or more, which has made me appreciate their existence all the more. We'll be together again soon.